THE
AROMATHERAPY COMPANION

MEDICINAL USES • AYURVEDIC HEALING • BODY CARE BLENDS
PERFUMES & SCENTS • EMOTIONAL HEALTH & WELL-BEING

VICTORIA H. EDWARDS

STOREY
BOOKS

*The mission of Storey Publishing is to serve our customers
by publishing practical information that encourages
personal independence in harmony with the environment.*

Edited by Deborah Balmuth
Writing assistance from Terry Meier
Cover design by Meredith Maker
Cover illustration by Laura Tedeschi
Text design and production by Susan Bernier
Herb illustrations and spot art by Laura Tedeschi
Line drawings by Alison Kolesar
Indexed by Indexes & Knowledge Maps

"A Bit of Botany" on page 25 is excerpted from the book *375 Essential Oils and Hydrosols* by Jeanne Rose, published by North Atlantic Books, 1999, and reproduced with the permission of the author.

Storey Books are available for special premium and promotional uses and for customized editions. For further information, please call Storey's Custom Publishing Department at 1-800-793-9396.

Printed in the United States by R.R. Donnelley
10 9 8 7 6 5 4 3

Library of Congress Cataloging-in-Publication Data

Edwards, Victoria H., 1949-
    The aromatherapy companion / Victoria H. Edwards.
      p.   cm.
    Includes index.
    ISBN 1-58017-150-8 (pbk. : alk. paper)
    1. Aromatherapy.   I. Title
  RM666.A68E39   1999
  615'.321—dc21
                                         99-26173
                                           CIP

Dedication

To my daughter, Cassandra Rose Edwards, my mother, Verna Ledet Hammer, and my faithful dog, Rosy.

Acknowledgments

My thanks go to many people: To Donovan L. Harmon, who was the first one to encourage me to write this book back in 1989; Marilyn Latyak for providing me a hideaway to get some writing done; Steve Bash, who reminded me to remember I am writing for my readers; Linda Kelleher, my faithful office manager; Terry Meier for the lioness's share of helping make my vague ideas more readable and knowing how to turn a sentence around and curtsy; Jeanne Rose, my mentor, who taught me a lot about botanical language and still continues to; Patrick Collins, who has made French aromatherapy come to life for me and generously taught at Aroma Camp in France; my editor Deborah Balmuth for her gentle strength and endurance; illustrators Laura Tedeschi and Alison Kolesar; and all the people at Storey Books who have worked on this book.

Contents

Preface

My dear gentle reader, it is for you that I stay up late into the night typing away, my eyes burning, barely able to see the liquid crystal screen. My intention has been to awaken you with the same inspiration and knowledge that I have gained along the scented path. For 14 years I have labored over this work. Longer than almost any painting, perfume blend, or other work of art.

My story begins when I was a girl of three, staying with my grandmother in Thibodaux, Louisiana. In my memories of my grandma, Eugenia Picou Ledet, her kitchen is always full of tastes and smells. I'll never forget the sight of headless chickens running around the big backyard. Who could? The vegetable garden was a necessity: It provided fresh tomatoes and okra to Mamie's seafood gumbos. If you've ever known any French people, then you know that fresh food and its scents are central to life itself.

The summer that I was four, I scratched my leg crawling under a barbed-wire fence and went crying to Mamie. She applied some homemade liniment. It smelled spicy and good; it burned at first, then soothed. I remember bright red hissing crabs trying to escape the boiling pot, and fresh pearly oysters in big burlap bags eaten "raw on the half shell" with horseradish. I recall the hot, sweet, bitter tastes of Louisiana. Coffee brewed with chicory and served in a demitasse cup with lots of sugar cubes. Toasted sugar, the best chocolate fudge, big fat pecan pralines on wax paper. At the family farm in the hot and humid bayou, I first tasted fresh raw sugarcane. My great-grandpa Ledet was a natural healer in the Cajun tradition.

I remember the smells from the bathroom cupboard, full of remedies like Dr. Tichenor's Thyme Liniment for mosquito bites and Dr Hausmann's Mexico Liniment, composed of spices including cloves, star anise, turkey rhubarb root, and peppermint. I loved baths in the deep old tub with its elaborate brass fixtures and the soft scent of Ivory soap and the faintest hint of lemongrass.

Mamie's bedroom dresser was full of bottles and little jars; sweet old Avon bottles, a blue deco Evening in Paris perfume bottle. I loved to smell the perfumes, the cedar chests, and the lavender sachets in the linen drawers. My journey upon the fragrant path had begun.

After my grandma died, her spirit came to visit me on her way to heaven. I was at the hospital, where I had just given birth to my daughter Cassandra. I awoke in the middle of the night and smelled her pale, powdery, vetiver scent. Mamie could still connect with me through fragrance, and she has been a spiritual guide for me ever since.

My botanical career also began around the age of four. I have fond memories of picking tiny wild purple pelargonium and storksbill, and concocting formulas in the old wooden garage out back.

My family moved to Germany just before my fifth birthday. My favorite pastime there was picking flowers on the hillsides. I picked honeysuckle to suck out its sweet juice, along with red clover blossoms, chamomile, sweet woodruff — in German, *der Waldemeister,* "master of the woods." I also enjoyed picking blueberries and collecting petrified wood.

Lilacs are so childlike and sweet when they are freshly picked. The smell of lilacs is my favorite, and a childhood memory of so many people I have met. Today I picked lilacs, and I marveled at their scent as they wilt — like little old ladies.

I invite you to join me for a walk along the scented path and share my lifelong enchantment with nature's gifts of ethereal scents and sublime colors. I am sure you will rediscover scent memories long ago forgotten. Just as a familiar song on the radio can evoke memories of times past, the scents of essential oils may stir up snapshot images of scenes and experiences from your earlier life. Please, walk with me along the pathways of your mind; come enjoy the fragrant journey.

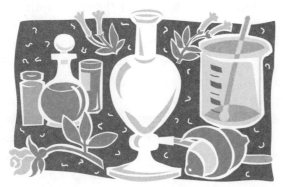

Introduction to Aromatherapy and Essential Oils

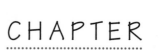

CHAPTER 1

In very simple terms, aromatherapy is the therapeutic use of pure essential oils to improve the health and balance of the skin, the body, the mind, and the soul.

Squeeze a lavender head or a sage leaf and smell your fingers. That aroma is the result of volatile oils, released by the bursting of tiny glands in the plant material. These volatile oils represent the radiant energy of the sun, translated by the plant into a chemical form. If you look at the same plant through a microscope, you will see the little pouches where these chemicals, the volatile oils, are stored. Although we don't yet fully understand the role these essential oils play in the drama of plants' life cycles, they have played a role throughout the development of human culture.

The quantity and quality of the essential oils that a plant produces depend on many things. Just as soil, elevation, and weather conditions; genus and species; horticulture, processing, and handling all influence the ultimate quality of a fine wine, so essential oils for therapeutic use vary according to the plants' conditions of growth.

WHAT ARE ESSENTIAL OILS?

Chemically, essential oils are a cocktail of molecules with names like esters, terpenes, alcohols, phenols, aldehydes, ketones, ethers, and sesquiterpenes, along with myriad other chemicals. These constituent parts have various properties. Some are anti-inflammatory, some antifungal, some antiviral, mucolytic, or bactericidal. All are antiseptic in varying degrees, and all are volatile. Essential oils fall naturally into three groups. The most highly volatile essential oils, known as *top notes* in the perfume industry, are those that evaporate most quickly. These oils tend to have an uplifting and invigorating action. Essential oils that have a lower volatility, and thus evaporate slowly, are known in the perfume industry as *bass notes.* These oils are most often used therapeutically for their calming and sedating

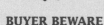

BUYER BEWARE

Imported essential oils are often cut or adulterated for the perfume industry, whose main concerns are price and aroma stability. Thus essential oil buying is not an easy task. A good importer of essential oils for aromatherapy must buy from many different sources and constantly test oils for purity.

action. And essential oils with a medium range of volatility, known as *middle notes* in perfumery, act to stimulate and regulate the main body systems.

Natural oils do not cause side effects when used properly. Essential oils have the power to relax the nervous system, stimulate the circulation, lift depression, reduce inflammation, and ease aches and pains. They can balance emotions by establishing harmony between the mind and body and lifting the conscious mind to the higher self. The aroma of an essential oil is sensed by the olfactory nerve located in the back of the nose and carried to the brain, where it has its effect — perhaps stimulating or calming, perhaps imparting feelings of well-being and harmony to the whole self.

Oils can also penetrate the skin's surface, and their benefits for the skin are profound. Essential oils can revitalize and rejuvenate skin of all ages and are especially helpful for skin problems such as acne, eczema, psoriasis, burns, scars, and even some skin cancers.

A professional aromatherapy treatment is usually combined with massage. Therapeutic and healing in itself, massage's effects are magnified when combined with aromatherapy. Massage can make us feel comforted and secure, because touch is an extension of our earliest memories; when combined with the appropriate essential oils, the benefits for mind and body are considerable.

Although many of the effects of essential oils have been proven through scientific research, their most profound healing qualities can only be observed. The effects of aromas on the psyche, along with their subtler effects of preventing illness, are difficult to measure. But aromatherapy represents one of the oldest healing arts known to mankind.

limbic system

smell sensory cortex

olfactory bulb

smell receptors

Scent sparks more of an emotional response than an intellectual one because of the direct impact it has on the limbic system, part of the most basic and primitive areas of our brain.

olfactory receptors

nasal cavity

path of air

When scent molecules hit the smell receptors in the nose, they set off impulse that travels along the nerves connected to the olfactory bulb (behind the eyes).

AROMATHERAPY THROUGH THE DAY

By incorporating aromatherapy into your daily routine, you can enjoy the natural health benefits of essential oils and aesthetically enhance previously humdrum activities.

Imagine waking to the invigorating scent of rosemary and basil drifting gently past your nose. It's not hard to achieve: Load a diffuser with a wake-up blend and plug into an automatic timer to start your day. In your morning shower, give your body an energizing loofah scrub with an aqua solution of thyme, savory, and tea tree. Follow your shower with a quick toweling, and then lock the residual moisture into your skin with a custom-designed body oil blend. You might add few drops of tea tree oil to the toothpaste on your toothbrush to help prevent gum disease and tooth decay.

On your way to work, place a tissue moistened with a drop of essential oil on the dashboard of your car to smooth out the drive. Along with your lipstick, carry a vial of peppermint oil: A drop on your tongue throughout the day will keep your breath fresh and help you stay alert. Before an important meeting, you might place a drop of rose oil on your tongue. It will give you confidence and create a loving atmosphere as the scent of rose is broadcast with your presentation. On your drive home a little clary sage on a tissue placed on your dashboard will help you unwind and cope with rush-hour traffic.

Later, an evening bath with chamomile, neroli, and marjoram will ensure a restful sleep. Or if you are cold, you might prefer a warming bath with black pepper, myrrh, sandalwood, Peru balsam, and ginger — Ahhh, another aromatic day.

What if you wake up feeling miserable? When everything hurts, when you've got the blues, cramps, or a headache, cancel your plans and take a hot steaming bath with eucalyptus, geranium, clary sage, and juniper. Make yourself a pot of herb tea and snuggle up in a warm bathrobe. You're sure to feel better soon.

THE ORIGINS OF AROMATHERAPY

The origins of aromatherapy lie hidden in the folds of time. Human-kind's earliest written documents record the use of plant oils for their healing and aesthetic properties. Ointments, oils, infusions, poultices, and incenses were all made from plants, and were the only medicines known until the late 19th century.

Ancient healers were holistic. They regarded healing as a transcendent art. From the same plants they used to heal the body, they derived perfumes to uplift the spirit, and they recognized these two actions as being different aspects of the same unifying plant energy. In contrast, modern science seeks to compartmentalize, and works to identify and separate plants' active constituents.

India

The people of India have always used infused fragrant matter for medicine and meditation. The Vedic literature of India, dating from around 2000 B.C., lists among its spiritual and healing substances cinnamon, spikenard, ginger, myrrh, coriander, sandalwood, patchouli, jasmine, and rose. The manner in which aromatics were viewed reflects a spiritual and philosophical outlook in which humanity is seen as a part of nature. In India aromatics are believed to be spiritual, and the handling of herbs and oils a sacred task. In the Indo-Aryan tongue, *attar* — which can mean "smoke," "wind," "odor," and "essence" — most often describes perfumed oil blends.

Attars of musk, hina, kewda, and champa have been used for thousands of years in India, primarily as components of Ayurvedic medicine (see chapter 10).

In traditional Indian weddings, kilos of flowers were once made into garlands and canopies and hung over the honeymoon bed. A beautiful Indian ritual, still practiced, is that of strewing flowers of frangipani, rose, tuberose, and jasmine on bedsheets to delight the senses.

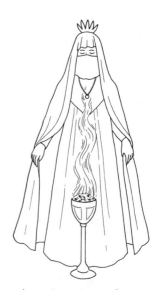

In ancient times, the aromatherapist used plant perfumes to heal the body and lift the emotions.

The *Kama Sutra*, a classic Indian treatise on lovemaking that includes poetically written detail on positions and practices, is filled with instructions for using various perfumes to fan the flames of love.

Classic Indian love potions were made with amber aged in wine, along with the essential oils of rose, sandalwood, frangipani, tuberose, hina, night queen, and the exotic floral scents of champa, mottia, and mogra.

BOTANICAL INCENSE

Incense is still used in the sacred rituals of the Roman Catholic and Eastern Orthodox Churches. The Western incense is composed of gum resins exuded from the bark of small trees, usually frankincense and myrrh, mixed with gum benzoin and sometimes rosemary oil. The mixture is sprinkled over burning charcoal in a censer (pictured).

Incense is also burned in Tibetan, Buddhist, and other temples all across the Eastern Hemisphere. In addition to frankincense and myrrh, Eastern perfumers use sandalwood, agarwood (oud), patchouli, and vetiver in formulating incense. The botanicals are ground to a paste with water, then created into elaborate shapes by pressing strings and coils through a perforated plate (much like a pasta press). Saltpeter or potassium nitrate is sometimes added to make the mixture burn steadily. In India, a simple incense is made by dipping joss sticks into oils.

Ancient China

"Every perfume is a medicine."

The use of five thousand different herbs, spices, and animal and mineral substances originated in China. Some of the important aromatherapy oils for which we have China to thank are cassia, star anise, angelica, camphor, musk, and ginger. Citrus trees also had their origins in China. In the 12th century Chang Shih-nan described placing orange blossoms in a burner and heating them until "drops of liquid collected like sweat." The distillate was poured over agarwood and kept in a porcelain jar to produce a fragrance of extraordinary elegance.

Chinese texts dating from as early as 3000 B.C. mention Shi-Che, the Chinese goddess of perfume, and describe the practices used to enhance the environment with scent. Sachets of perfumed powders were tucked into voluminous sleeves; perfume burners and joss sticks scented every room. Prunings of aromatic tree barks were kept in laundry, and paper strips were impregnated with perfume, with bits torn off and carried for their scent. At one time Chinese money was printed on silk and perfumed. The Oriental philosophy was to perfume the environment rather than the person.

Ancient Babylon and Egypt

The first perfumes in Egypt were aromatics kindled as incense to the gods. Incense was burned at all important events, including the opening of a shrine, the coronation of a pharaoh, and national celebrations. The cloud of aromatic smoke exuded by incense created an aura that was believed to attract good influences and repel negative spirits.

Incense was burned daily in ancient Egyptian temples, and outdoors at dusk and dawn. The Papyrus of Ebers includes descriptions of the use of aromatics for magical, mystical, and healing experiences.

EARLY ALCHEMIST

Maria Prophetissima was an alchemist who lived in Alexandria, Egypt, during the first century A.D. At this time, Alexandria was rife with exploration and experimentation. Egyptians were developing new art forms and techniques in metallurgy, glassmaking, jewelry, ceramics, and perfumery. Maria studied many of these arts. She created the first true still, a covered post whose vapors could waft out. Her contraption, which she called a *kerotakis*, was intended, in her own words, "to enable the alchemist to find the essence of that which is bodily, and embody that which is spirit."

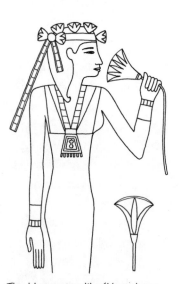

The blue water lily (*Nymphaea caerulea*) was one of the best-loved plants in ancient Egyptian culture, for both its fragrance and its intoxicating properties. Cleopatra, the last of the Egyptian queens, was noted for her use of scent and oils. The story of her first meeting with Mark Antony is legendary: She is said to have soaked the sails of her barge in perfume, scented her gowns with the finest perfumes, and surrounded herself with a cloud of aromatic incense as she sat on her throne, floating up the Nile to greet and seduce Mark Antony.

Incense was employed in exorcisms and healing the sick; it was used ritually in lovemaking. The smoke was believed to honor and please the gods and bring good luck. It was believed that incense smoke had the power to attract heavenly beings, so that those who had died and were beyond the reach of the living might survive, their souls ascending on a cloud of smoky aroma.

Early Egyptian priests practiced enfleurage, an extraction process obtaining aromatic oils from flowers (see page 15). The first cosmetics were composed of resins, myrrh, frankincense, lilies, pine, cedar, gum mastic, mints, and terebinth and stored in elegant containers of carved onyx, alabaster, ivory, obsidian, and glass decorated with gold.

Egypt is still a major producer of essential oils. Some of the important aromatherapy oils exported from Egypt are rose, jasmine, neroli, violet leaf, geranium, petitgrain, basil, marjoram, anise, and parsley seed.

The Ancient Mideast

The most prized of all incenses to the Mesopotamians was the fragrant cedar-of-Lebanon *(Cedrus libani)*. The name "Lebanon" comes from the Akkadian word *lubbunu,* which means "incense." King Solomon's Temple was built twice of fragrant cedar-of-Lebanon trees. After being destroyed in 586 B.C., the temple was rebuilt in 535 B.C. with the aid of the Persians, again using fragrant cedarwood.

Ancient Greece

The Greeks originally learned about aromatic oils from the Egyptians. Crete had an elegant culture that lasted from 2600 to 1250 B.C. Phoenician ships carried Cretan rhyton vessels to Egypt and returned with items made in Egypt, including aromatic oils.

Greeks ascribed a divine origin to all aromatic plants. Dionysus was the god of scent, flavor, wine, and perfume. He bestowed blessings and scents on flowers. Cloris was the deity of flowers, and Eros is an anagram for *rose.* At Delphi, the virgin priestesses were anointed with and bathed in oils.

Hippocrates, 460–377 B.C., known as the Father of Modern Medicine, identified disease as a natural phenomenon, and for the first time established a system of diagnosis and prognosis. He acquired most of his knowledge from Egyptian sources. He used about four hundred drugs, derived mainly from botanicals. Hippocrates is said to have saved Athens from the Plague by setting huge bonfires of aromatic wood in the streets.

Theophrastus of Eresus, 372–287 B.C., was a friend and pupil of Aristotle. He wrote the *Historia Plantarum* as well as the first treatise on scent, "Concerning Odors." He took an elaborate inventory of all known aromatics and discussed ways in which they could be artfully blended. He considered the properties of the oils used as carriers of scent, scents infused in wines, and the influence of various perfumes on states of mind and health.

Dioscorides, a Greek physician in the first century A.D., was without a doubt the first real medical botanist. A physician with the Roman army, he assembled one vast work, *De Materia Medica,* that described more than six hundred plants, including their habitats, medicinal effects, and preparations. For 1,500 years his *Materia Medica* set the standard for herbal knowledge.

Ancient Rome

The Romans exceeded all limits in their outrageous and lavish use of aromatic substances.

Along with bathing, they adopted the sumptuous use of aromatics as a social form of amusement and entertainment. Built into the

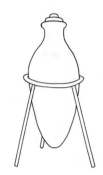

Ancient Greeks stored aromatic oils in amphoras, ceramic vessels that were buried in the sand to protect the oils from sun and heat.

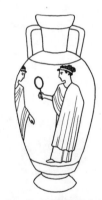

The Greeks crafted elaborate ceramic perfumery jars to store their valued fragranced oils.

walls of their colossal bathhouses were shelves specially designed to hold the decorative vessels that contained aromatic unguents. Matrons were massaged and bathed in perfumes by slaves called *cosmetae*. The *aromatarii* were the perfumers of Rome, and they lived in a special section of the city called the *vicus thuraricus.*

Some of the components of Roman perfumery during the height of decadence were roses, iris (orrisroot), narcissus, saffron, mastic, oakmoss, cinnamon, cardamon, nutmeg, ginger, costus, spikenard, aloeswood, fragrant grasses, and gum resins.

Pliny the Elder was the most important writer on plants in ancient Rome. In A.D. 77 he composed his *Historia Naturalis* (Natural History). Of the 37 volumes, 7 were on plants. Pliny wrote that scent could lull a person to sleep, allay anxiety, and brighten dreams. He recorded the names of two perfumes: Mendes, named for a town famous for its fragrances, and Kyphi, which means "welcome to the Gods." The latter, compounded of cypress, juniper, incense, resins, hina, mint, sweet flag, and aromatic grasses, is one of the world's most enduring perfume blends.

Pliny recorded a fatal case of flower gluttony that occurred in Imperial Rome under Nero's reign. Banquet guests were actually smothered to death when volumes of rose petals were dropped upon them. Pliny used this example to decry the abuse of perfumes by the citizens of Rome.

Medieval Arabia: Home of the Damask Rose

Persia's use of aromatics is one of the most ancient, but unfortunately few of the culture's documents have been translated. Arabians are credited with the development of steam distillation, as well as true soapmaking. Avicenna, a Persian physician, was for centuries thought to be the first to practice steam distillation. (The process has now been dated to earlier periods based on excavated pottery found in newer archaeological digs.) He did, however, invent the refrigerated coil, and is the first person known to have distilled rose oil. Avicenna was a prodigy, practicing medicine at the age of 18. He used pulse diagnosis and generously prescribed the use of all parts of the rose: leaf and petal, rose jam, rose water, rose hips, and essence of rose.

Saudi Arabia and Oman are still the center of precious resin production.

Europe

Give me an ounce of civet, good apothecary, to sweeten my imagination.

— Shakespeare

France has a very richly scented history. Cave paintings in Lascaux illustrate the Neanderthals' use of medicinal plants. Perfume sellers were recorded in Paris as early as 1190. Catherine de Medici made Paris the city of perfume when she arrived in 1533 to marry Henry II. Catherine brought along her own perfumer, Rene, who established his famous shop, decorated with an Egyptian motif, on the Pont au Change. The Medici family, wealthy and powerful in Italy, were famous for their clever poison rings and perfumed gloves. Nostradamus, whose prophetic skill is extolled to this day, was a perfumer and alchemist as well as Catherine's astrologer.

France's monarchs were said to be the "sweetest smelling." Eau d'Hongrie, or Hungary Water, created in 1370 for the queen of Hungary, was originally a "Plague water" meant to keep disease at bay. Eau de Cologne and Acqua Perata were other perfumes that originated as curatives. Eau de Cologne is a blend of attar of neroli, orange, rosemary, and bergamot.

Napoleon was notoriously neurotic about scent. Preserved receipts document his routine purchases of huge quantities of eau de Cologne. He is said to have used the perfume especially heavily when going into battle to give the men in his troops confidence in his leadership.

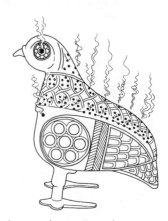

Incense burners, such as this partridge-shaped container, were an art form in 12th century Persia.

WELCOMING SCENTS
It was a custom throughout the ancient Orient to honor guests by anointing them with oils and rose water.

In a famous letter to his beloved Josephine he commanded, "Don't wash, I'll be home in a few weeks." Napoleon disliked the popular scent of musk, and after he betrayed her with another woman, Josephine spitefully had his bed chamber sprayed with musk, an odor that is said to cling forever.

Contemporary Aromatherapy

Medicine, perfumery, and herbalism trod the same path until well into the 19th century, but diverged in the latter half of the 1800s. With the advent of modern chemistry and a general infatuation with science, traditional medicines came to be considered primitive, and the public adopted the belief that anything created or tinkered with in the laboratory must be superior to the "raw" material. With the invention of synthetics, perfumery set off in an altogether different direction as scent came to be associated with a burgeoning cosmetic market.

Today's rediscovery of the wonderful healing properties of essential oils is largely due to the French chemist Rene Maurice Gattefossé. He found, during World War I (1910), that lavender had a profound healing effect on burns, and went on to make the study of the healing properties of essential oils his life's work. In 1937 Gattefossé wrote his groundbreaking *Aromatherapie: Les Huiles essentielles, hormons vegetales.* In it he pointed out "the large number of aromatic substances that can be used in medicine and the wide variety of their chemical functions," and noted "two properties are common to them all: they are *volatile* and they are *aromatic.*"

Since then France has continued to be a hotbed of aroma research. It has expanded the use of essential oils beyond perfumery and cosmetics, into commerce and medicine.

Germany is one European country that has always maintained its reliance on the herbal tradition, marrying herbal use with science quite well. Today Germany excels in the latest scientific analysis of essential oils and in the development of new testing technology.

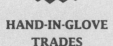

HAND-IN-GLOVE TRADES

The *peau d'Espana* (skin of Spain) was a goatskin bag carried from Morocco to France in the 1400s. It was "cured" in rose oil to heal it from a rotting disease. This event marked the beginning of a long association between the arts of perfumery and glove making. The two trades evolved simultaneously from the curing of hides — perfume was used to hide the scent of the urine used in curing. By the 18th century, many glove makers had turned exclusively to perfumery.

HOW ESSENTIAL OILS ARE MADE

Although the term *essential oil* is commonly used to refer to any oil extracted from a plant, a "true" essential oil is one that has been collected through steam distillation. The French consider steam-distilled oils the only true essential oils, and the only ones worthy of use in aromatherapy. Other means of extraction exist, however, and the resulting products, named accordingly, have found a place in popular aromatherapy.

Steam Distillation

The traditional method of extracting essential oils — steam distillation — remains the most widely used method of production throughout the world. Steam distillation works effectively because of the high volatility and insolubility of essential oils.

A simple steam-distillation still consists of a covered vat connected to a receiver vessel through a tube or "coil." The vat, a large cylindrical metal tank, is filled with water and plant material and covered with a special lid called the "col de cygne" (swan neck). Heat is applied and, as the water boils, steam passes through the plant material and evaporates the oils. The col de cygne collects the steam and directs it through the attached tube or coil, which is "refrigerated" with running water. The steam condenses and drips into the receiver vessel or "vase Florentine" (Florentine vase), where the mixture of condensed water and oil separates naturally. Depending on its density, the essential oil will either float above or come to rest beneath the water.

A delightful by-product of steam distillation, called hydrosol or hydrolate, is created as the water becomes impregnated with the aroma of the plant being distilled. Floral waters such as rose water and orange water are well-known examples of hydrosols. (See chapter 6 for more on hydrosols.)

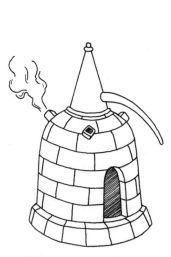

A 16th century distillation still.

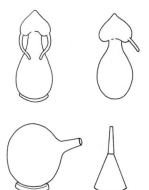

17th century alchemist's equipment used for extracting essential oils.

Essential Oil Extraction Processes

Process	Product
Steam distillation	Essential oil
Manual extraction	Pressed oil
Enfleurage	Concrète
Maceration	Concrète
Solvent extraction	Absolute
Critical carbon dioxide	CO_2 oil
Phytonic	Florasol
Laboratory synthesis	Fragrance oil

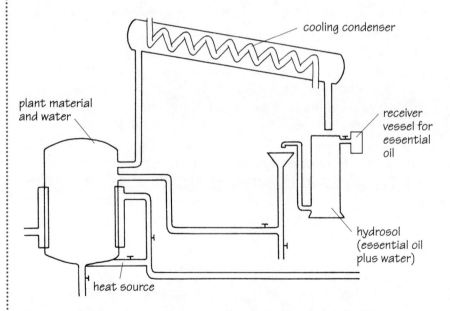

In steam distillation, plant material is combined with water in the large tank (at bottom left). When the water boils, the oils evaporate, are collected, and run through a cooling condenser. As they cool, the essential oils separate from the water and drip into the receiving vessel.

Manual Extraction

Manual extraction yields pressed oils. *Pressed oil* is a term applied exclusively to oils from the citrus family. The essential oils in citrus reside in tender chambers just below the surface of the rind. As the rind is torn, the tiny chambers are broken and the volatile oils leap out. You have no doubt, while peeling an orange, felt the sudden sharp sting of citrus oil hit your eye. You can observe the wild antics of freshly released citrus oils by pressing the peel of a lemon or an orange in front of a candle flame. The volatile oils become visible as they ignite in tiny flashes upon contact with the flame.

The traditional manual-extraction method calls for plunging your bare hands into a tub of citrus rinds and grabbing and squeezing vigorously to break the oil globules and release the essential oils. As the oil separates from the resulting mush, it rises to the surface and can be collected with a sponge. The oil-saturated sponge can then be squeezed into a separate container.

Although this process is still used, these days the squeezing is more often accomplished mechanically.

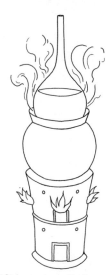

An 18th century Italian distillation system.

Enfleurage

Enfleurage, which yields a concrète, is a very old method of extracting aromatic oils from flowers. It is especially effective with delicate tropical flowers that tend to break down rapidly or become spoiled in the heat of distillation.

Enfleurage is begun by placing flowers on a sheet of glass that has been prepared by being coated with a thick layer of purified fat. The flowers are replaced with fresh ones daily, and the process is repeated until the fat has become saturated with essential oil and the desired concentration is obtained. The resultant compound is called a concrète. If the waxes are left in and it is used in this state as an ointment or perfume, it is called a pomade.

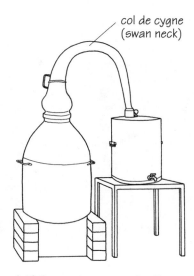

col de cygne
(swan neck)

A 19th century copper distillation unit.

Enfleurage is still used as a method of extraction, but is usually carried to its second stage — dissolving the concrète in alcohol. Although fat is insoluble in alcohol, essential oil readily dissolves in it. The resulting liquid is then carefully heated; as the alcohol evaporates, the pure essential oil is left in the container. This is what is referred to as an absolute.

Maceration

Maceration is similar to enfleurage but easily performed in your kitchen. Start with a very clean, empty glass jar, a knife or scissors, and your hands. Find some aromatic plant material; rosemary or basil will work quite well. As you break up and crush the flowers or leaves, the oil cells will rupture, releasing the plant material's aromatic properties.

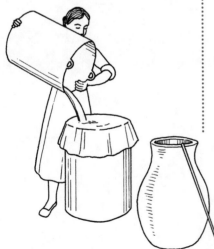

Maceration, soaking crushed plant material in olive oil, produces a concrète when strained.

Place the crushed plant material in the jar and cover it with vegetable oil you have warmed to the temperature of a baby's bath; olive or almond oil is a good choice (you can also use purified fat).

Place the jar outside in the sun or another warm place. The optimum length of time for soaking really depends on the material and the climate. To produce the popular red oil from St.-John's-wort flowers, the traditional Greek method calls for 21 days of soaking, while the French prescribe three months. I have found, however, that in very warm weather, two days can be too much! So experiment. As the vegetable oil or fat absorbs aroma, strain off the old plant material and submerge a fresh batch into your rewarmed carrier base. Repeat the process until the vegetable oil or fat has reached the desired concentration.

If you use vegetable oil, the resulting liquid is good in massage treatments or in homemade herbal creams. With fat you can use the resulting pomade, or treat it as in the second stage of enfleurage.

Solvent Extraction

Oils produced through solvent extraction are also called absolutes. In simple terms, the flowers are covered with a solvent (usually petrol ether), which extracts the essential oil. The solvent is then evaporated off, leaving the essential oil in the container.

Solvent-extracted oils are becoming suspect. Solvents are unkind chemicals that threaten our environment. Traces of solvent can also be left behind, resulting in an unpleasant product. I prefer to avoid them when possible.

Critical Carbon Dioxide

Critical carbon dioxide (CO_2) and subcritical are two of the most contemporary methods of extraction. These cold processes are able to capture the purest and finest notes. Oils produced with these methods are called cold-processed CO_2 oils or subcritical oils; they are superior oils that retain extremely delicate notes usually lost in steam distillation. CO_2 and subcritical oils have the fragrance of a freshly picked plant.

These methods were developed in the 1950s, in the search for a process that would eliminate the contamination and degradation found with conventional solvent extraction and steam distillation.

The process of extraction with liquid carbon dioxide requires a great deal of expensive equipment. Under extremely high pressure and extremely low temperatures, carbon dioxide becomes a liquid solvent capable of extracting essential oils while avoiding the thermal degradation associated with distilling at atmospheric pressure.

CO_2 and subcritical essential oils are very delicate. They should be kept in full, dark glass bottles in a cool, dark place.

The Phytonic Process

Also known as Wilde's Process or Peter's Process, the phytonic process is an exciting development in plant oil extraction technology. Invented in the late 1980s by Dr. Peter Wilde of Sowerby Thirsk, England, this process results in what's called a florasol or phytol.

The phytonic process uses a hydrofluorocarbon solvent (HFC 134a), which is injected into a sealed unit containing the aromatic plant material. After a period of contact between the solvent — a liquefied gas — and the plant material, at room temperature, a solution of oil is formed. The solution is released into another sealed chamber, where it is allowed to gently evaporate at temperatures well below freezing. The entire solvent gas is recovered, collected, and reliquefied for reuse. What remains is a pure florasol containing a full complement of delicate aromatic components along with a small percentage of moisture. The quality of the florasol is exquisite, with a remarkably fresh and pure scent.

Although HFCs are considered a serious threat to the environment, Dr. Wilde assures me that his process is environmentally sound and safe to use, because the small amount of HFC is recycled and never released into the atmosphere. Several industrial-scale plants are currently using this process.

Compared to other procedures, the phytonic process uses less energy, produces no flue gases or residual toxic waste, uses no water or heat, and works at room temperature. I believe this process may be poised to displace the more expensive and damaging methods currently in use.

Dr. Wilde has also developed and demonstrated small handheld "jungle kits." These kits, about the size of a baby's bottle, can be carried into the field for on-the-spot extractions. I used one of these at a workshop in France and personally experienced the healing power of the resulting florasol, when I applied fresh lavender extract to a badly bruised and skinned leg. My skin healed rapidly.

SYNTHETIC OILS

Coal comes from deep within the earth, the result of layers of decomposing plant material subjected over millions of years to great heat and pressure. Coke, a derivative of coal that burns with intense heat and produces very little smoke, became an important fuel during the Industrial Revolution. It is produced by burning coal in airtight ovens. Coal tar is a thick, black, viscous by-product of coke production. Originally a nuisance, coal tar has become the mainstay of the modern chemical industry. Countless synthetic compounds have been developed from it, including dyes, fragrances, and explosives.

Until the mid-1800s, however, coal tar was rather unappreciated. Composed almost wholly of carbon and hydrogen, it didn't burn easily and was fairly resistant to most chemical and oxidizing agents. The coal tar deadlock was broken with the discovery that a combination of sulfuric and nitric acids could break down its carbon and hydrogen. As coal tar derivatives were treated with chemicals, the result was myriad new products. One we are all familiar with is nitrobenzene, or false oil of bitter almonds, which is used to scent floor wax, cleaning products, and shoe polish. You might be familiar with nitrobenzene as the scent of Jergens Lotion.

Redesigning Nature

Within a few short years of the coal tar breakthrough, Friedrich August Kekulé (1829–1896) founded modern structural chemistry. According to legend, while riding in a form of public transportation of the time, he fell asleep and missed his stop. This annoyance was compensated for, however, by a dream in which carbon atoms joined hands and danced around him in a circle. It was this dream that Kekulé claimed as his inspiration for the creation of structural chemistry.

AROMATIC ENDING
Alexander the Great used aromatics quite sumptuously. His funeral pyre was built of aromatic resins.

Kekulé envisioned not only deconstructing substances, as coal tar chemistry had achieved, but also reconstructing and even rearranging carbon atoms to create new substances. Carbon is the main component of several million known compounds and has the unusual ability to combine not only with other atoms but with itself as well. Carbon has a tremendous capacity for organizing and structuring matter, and its capacity for reorganization makes for a huge number of possible combinations.

Some of these combinations would imitate substances in nature. Voilà: The era of synthetics had arrived. Sweet-tasting substances were synthesized and put into production. A whole range of synthetic dyes became commercially available. And ingenious synthesizing also yielded an abundance of artificial scents, each imitating a different plant fragrance.

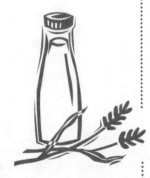

Synthetics versus Natural Oils

Synthetic oils, or oils blended with synthetic substances, however pleasant they may smell, are unacceptable for use in aromatherapy. A synthetic fragrance is a dead product and has no place in holistic aromatherapy. Synthetics should never be used for healing, strengthening, or health-promoting purposes. They have no healing properties. On the contrary, they may endanger your health. Synthetics can set off allergic reactions and tax your immune system. Central nervous system damage has been linked to the use of synthetic substances.

Synthetic oils and blends are never considered pure. They can contain by-products that are not easily identified, and their effects are unpredictable. Synthetics are listed as "fragrances" on most labels. Fragrances lack the vital energy that is responsible for the positive, healing effect of pure essential oils on mind and body.

Adulteration

The high price of pure essential oil accounts for much of the mixing and diluting referred to as "blending" in the aroma industry. While the price for a quart of synthetic jasmine oil ranges between $8 and $50, a quart of pure essential oil of jasmine will cost closer to $2,000.

Terms such as *cutting, diluting, bouqueting,* and *rounding off* are all poor attempts to disguise the cruel truth: adulteration. Certain suppliers with highly developed imaginations will even use the term *ennobling* to describe the disfiguring of an essential oil.

Unfortunately, there exists a long history of mishandling natural oils, mislabeling them, and fraudulent sales of them to unsuspecting buyers. The pioneers of aromatherapy in the United States have fought this standard practice for years. Finally, with the recent advent of reliable testing by independent laboratories, we have become able to expose such unethical practices. Distributors who force essential oil suppliers to prove authenticity through chemical analysis are leading the way to a greater number of safer products for the consumer.

Unfortunately, your first exposure to aromatic oils is likely to be to synthetics. Synthetic fragrances are inexpensive and easily available. I will never forget one of my early experiences with synthetic oils. I was a teenager, enthralled with the romance of scent. On a hot, sultry summer day I rubbed some inexpensive, sweetly scented frangipani oil on my neck. Imagine my alarm when my neck broke out in an itchy, bumpy red rash that remained for the rest of the day. This was long before I knew that aromatherapy existed.

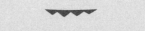

UNFRIENDLY ADDITIVES

Some of the chemicals and synthetics that are used as diluents to stretch oils and increase profits are:

- diethyl phthalate or DEP
- dipropylene glycol or DPG
- isopropyl myristate or IPM
- phenyl ethyl alcohol or PEA
- butylated hydroxy toluene or BHT (neurotoxic)

According to an alarming EPA report released in 1991, BHT was detected in every fragrance sample collected for study.

Many of the chemicals found in fragrances are also designated as hazardous waste chemicals. These include methylene chloride, toluene, methyl ethyl ketone, methyl isobutyl ketone, ethanol, and benzyl chloride.

Over the last 15 years I have been engaged in the worldwide commerce of essential oils. I have met wonderful people and learned a lot about quality. I've also observed shockingly unethical business practices and smelled a lot of stinking product. Although I trust my nose and my intuition, I have learned to request samples and chemical analyses from independent laboratories before purchasing oils from companies I'm not familiar with.

HEALTH COMPLAINTS MOST FREQUENTLY ASSOCIATED WITH FRAGRANCES

According to the FDA, fragrances are responsible for 30 percent of all allergic reactions to cosmetics. The Candida Research and Information Foundation (CRIF) of Castro Valley, California, surveyed some 10,000 physicians, patients, and health food store customers. The foundation's goal is mandatory removal of all neurotoxic chemicals from perfumes. Its findings indicated that the health complaints most frequently associated with fragrances and synthetic perfumes are:

- Headache
- Spaciness
- Inability to concentrate
- Mood changes
- Nausea
- Depression
- Sleepiness
- Sinus problems
- Restlessness, agitation
- Short-term memory lapse

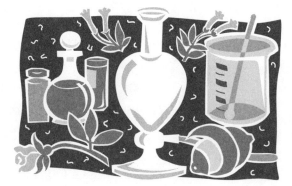

An Overview of
Essential Oils
and Their
Properties

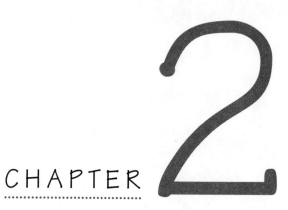

CHAPTER 2

Known as polyvalents (effective against many toxins), seven essential oils are applicable to many common ailments: lavender, geranium, eucalyptus, rosemary, lemon, cypress, and peppermint. These are the oils that are most frequently discussed in magazine articles and books about aromatherapy, and most often presented in aromatherapy seminars and classes. They are the oils most readily available for purchase, and the ones most often included in aromatherapy kits. Of the hundreds of essential oils being produced around the world today, it is no coincidence that these seven are the most frequently used.

LAVENDER (*Lavandula angustifolia*)

Any introduction to aromatherapy must begin with lavender oil. Simple and safe to use, lavender and its prolific offspring lavandin (produced from hybrids) are the most versatile of essential oils.

Lavender grows in clumps about 3 feet (90 cm) high, with long, thin, grayish green leaves and spikes of purple blossom clusters about 3 inches (7.5 cm) long. Both the flowers and the leaves have aromatic properties, and both parts of the plant are used in the distillation process.

Wild lavender (*Lavandula angustifolia* ssp. *angustifolia*), a plant with narrower leaves, produces an exquisite oil, and is considered to have more healing properties than any other type of lavender. Oil from the wild variety, however, has nearly disappeared from the marketplace, due to the extraordinary effort required to produce it. Native to the high mountains of southern France, the Canary Islands, and Persia, wild lavender grows on rocky, barren slopes where few other plants are able to survive the intense heat of summer and the bitter cold of winter. To harvest the hardy perennial, wildcrafters travel high up into the mountains in search of the choicest lavender. They pick during the hottest time of day, when

---

**THE SENSATIONAL
SEVEN OILS**

Lavender
Geranium
Eucalyptus
Rosemary
Lemon
Cypress
Peppermint

the essential oil content is at its peak, and carry their harvest, bundled on their backs, down into the valleys for distillation.

For commercial use, the higher-yielding species of lavender are cultivated and account for most of the true lavender oil available today.

A BIT OF BOTANY

Genus is the Latin term for "kind." We use the word to describe a group of closely related species. In botanical nomenclature, a plant's genus is always listed first, in italics, with the first letter capitalized.

Species refers to a particular form or kind, and is usually the smallest unit in a classification of organisms. A species is usually a group of individuals of the same ancestry, of nearly identical structure and behavior, and of relative stability in nature. The individuals of a species ordinarily interbreed freely and maintain their characteristics in nature.

A subspecies is a subdivision within a species. The term is usually used to designate a morphological group whose members are wholly, or at least partially, isolated geographically.

Variety as a botanical term can be employed in several senses. It is widely used to describe a morphologically distinct group, occupying a restricted area. The emphasis is on the small-scale, more localized range of a variety, compared to the large-scale regional basis of a subspecies. The variety designation is also used to describe variations whose precise nature is not understood, a treatment often necessary in the pioneer phase of taxonomy.

Chemotype is a term used to describe the chemical composition of an essential oil in which one chemical constitutent dominates. A chemotype is usually a result of a particular terroir.

Terroir is a French word that has infiltrated aromatherapy. It means the expression of the earth, or the particular planting site, in the resultant essential oil. Terroir is a factor of soil, shade, wind, water, rain, and terrain.

—Jeanne Rose

Legendary Lavender

Throughout history lavender has been recognized and appreciated for its calming qualities. It was commonly used by the classical Greeks and Romans, who perfumed their bathwater with lavender, burned lavender incense to appease their wrathful gods, and believed the scent of lavender to be soothing to untamed lions and tigers. To this day, many North African women wear lavender, believing it will prevent cruel treatment from their husbands.

Lavender has also played a premier role in herbal lore. Hildegard von Bingen, a Catholic nun, activist, and noted 12th-century herbalist, listed lavender's virtues: "[It is] especially good for all forms of headache and migraine, as a restorative and tonic against weakness, spasms, giddiness, colic and vertigo. It causes melancholy to go away and raises the spirits. A drop or two in a glass of water is a good gargle to hoarseness and loss of voice."

LAVENDER STILLS

For hundreds of years, making lavender oil was an annual ritual throughout southeastern France. Until the turn of the 20th century, most farms in the area had their own distillation equipment. These small stills were used for the extraction of essential oils (mostly wild lavender) in summer and for the fabrication of brandy in winter. In some parts of Provence and the Roussillon area of France, every village still has at least one distillery.

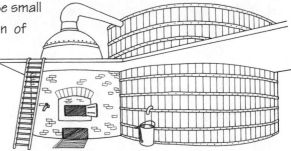

This 19th century still was typical of the units used in France to distill large amounts of lavender essential oil.

Gattefossé, the father of modern aromatherapy, experimented widely with lavender oil in 1910. He found it beneficial to the brain, nerves, paralysis, lethargy, and rheumatism, calming to the skin and muscles, useful in treating cold and flu, and safe enough for use on young children and pregnant women.

Therapeutic Uses

Lavender oil is employed as an aromatic, a carminative (soothing to the digestive system), and a nervine (soothing to the nervous system). Its healing power is due to a complex variety of chemical constituents (160 different components have been identified in the oil). Conditions to which lavender oil is applicable include depression, insomnia, stress, hoarseness, headache, burns, acne, sore muscles, sprains, stiff joints, nervous tension, hair loss, and childbirth.

Lavandin (*Lavandula* x *intermedia)* a hybrid of lavender that gives a high yield of a different quality essential oil resembling true lavender, is often sold as lavender oil. Although lavandin's properties and uses are similar to those of true lavender, it often has a higher proportion of camphor, giving a sharper, less pleasant smell. Lavandin is also less sedative than true lavender. As an alternative to true lavender, lavandin is useful as an inhalation for colds and congestion, as a bath or massage oil for muscle pain and stiffness, or for any condition for which lavender's camphorous qualities are indicated.

***Lavare:* "to wash."** With a name taken from the Latin word *lavare,* lavender is the premier oil for bathing, soothing, and disinfecting. It is an excellent choice for hair, scalp, and skin care, as a bath oil, and as a douche ingredient. One drop of lavender in a cup (235 ml) of water makes an antiseptic lavender water (not to be confused with lavender hydrosol, a by-product of distillation) that is soothing and cleansing for wounds or acne. Lavender water can be used as a wash for puffy eyes, bruises, bites, and other minor external sores, and as a hair rinse to reduce oiliness. Blended with

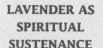

LAVENDER AS SPIRITUAL SUSTENANCE

The fragrance of lavender is said to open the Third Eye, and induce clairvoyance and inner vision. It brings light when our nervous system is agitated, overexcited, and overwrought. Lavender eases loneliness and offers emotional warmth. It is used in affirmations to relax nervous conditions. Lavender, used in meditation, assists visualizing purple-violet, a color associated in metaphysics with our pituitary and pineal gland, also called the master gland.

chamomile, bergamot, and neroli, and diluted in a carrier oil, lavender is beneficial for treating eczema and psoriasis. A few drops of lavender oil blended with basil or rosemary oil and brushed into hair promotes healthy growth.

Add 5 to 20 drops of lavender oil to a tub of water for a soothing bath. For a fresh and clean feeling when you are hot and tired, wipe your face and neck with a few drops of lavender on a wet washcloth.

Blending Lavender

Lavender blends well with, and its properties are enhanced by, other oils such as bergamot, geranium, clary sage, and rosemary. Blended with chamomile or rose, lavender retains a very soft and gentle character. Lavender blended with eucalyptus or geranium is stimulating to the immune system. Lavender oil, for application to any inflammation, should always be blended in a 1 percent concentration with water, an odorless cream base, or a vegetable or nut oil.

GERANIUM (*Pelargonium spp.*)

Geranium oil is prepared from the leaves and stalks of the scented geranium, *Pelargonium*. Of the many species in the *Pelargonium* genus, the oil is most often derived from the *P.* x *asperum* and *P. graveolens*.

Therapeutic Uses

The active ingredients in geranium oil are geraniol, geranyl acetate, and citronellol. The oil has a calming, balancing, and uplifting effect, making it a helpful treatment for depression, nervous anxiety, and fear. It acts as an excellent adrenal support, treating exhaustion, and its hormone-regulating properties make it especially applicable during puberty, menses, and menopause.

ORIGINS OF GERANIUM

Distilled primarily in Egypt and the islands of Bourbon and Comoro, geranium oil is clear and light green, with a beautifully fresh aroma and a relaxing and balancing effect. Geranium oil is also produced in China, although the Chinese variety, more orange in color, has a less refined scent than the African varieties.

Geranium oil is antioxidant, antiseptic, and astringent, and has been used as a treatment for wounds and ulcers. It is also effective in treating yeast-related ailments such as candida and athlete's foot.

Geranium oil makes a refreshing bath oil, and combines well with oils of rose, citrus, and basil. It can be used in all types of cosmetic preparations and is very effective whenever an astringent is called for. Geranium oil is balancing for both oily and dry complexions, and is helpful in treating acne and aging skin. It is an effective ingredient for treating skin disorders such as eczema and shingles. Added to massage oils, geranium is a deterrent to the herpes virus.

A mild rinse made by adding 1 drop of geranium oil to a cup (235 ml) of water is especially soothing to sores in the mouth and on the tongue. Geranium hydrosol (a by-product of the distillation process, not to be confused with an oil-water mixture) can be used to soothe conjunctivitis (inflammation of the mucous membrane surrounding the eye). Rose geranium oil has properties similar to geranium and can be used as a substitute.

EUCALYPTUS (Eucalyptus globulus)

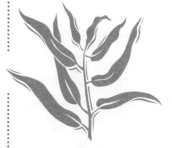

Native to Australia, eucalyptus are among the tallest trees in the world. Eucalyptus oil is most commonly extracted from the green branches, leaves, and nuts of the species *E. globulus,* which reaches heights of up to 200 feet (61 m). One of the world's fastest-growing trees, but sensitive to cold and frost, the eucalyptus has been introduced to many tropical and semitropical areas of the world. Commercial growth and oil production is still primarily in Australia.

Therapeutic Uses

Eucalyptus oil has widespread application. As an especially effective expectorant, it is the most common cough, cold, and sinus remedy throughout the world. The primary component of eucalyptus oil, present in concentrations ranging from 59 to 75 percent, is an oxide identified as 1,8 cineol. This cineol oxide (commonly known as eucalyptol) is the highly valued active ingredient in countless cough drops, elixirs, balms, salves, and suppositories.

Eucalyptus oil, inhaled or rubbed on the chest, helps clear congested respiratory passages. This treatment is beneficial for all respiratory tract infections, sinusitis, coughs, and sore throats as well as typhoid fever, tuberculosis, and malaria. Eucalyptus oil is used in the bath for its antiseptic action and employed in massage oils and ointments to treat chapped hands, lips, and other skin irritations. In combination with juniper and lavender, eucalyptus makes an effective rub for painful joints and muscles.

A drop of eucalyptus oil on a sugar cube or absorbed in honey and taken with water or tea has a strong antiseptic and diuretic effect on the urinary tract, is healing to the bladder, and is helpful for colds, herpes, flu, or other viral infections. The complete eucalyptus oil is more effective against infections than the isolated compound eucalyptol.

OTHER VARIETIES OF EUCALYPTUS OIL

E. radiata has an extremely soft fragrance and gentle effect. It is an excellent choice for inhalations. To purify and heal a room of sickness or negative, conflicting energies, diffuse into the room.

E. dives is excellent for skin infections, acne, and more.

E. smithii is less effective for respiratory problems.

E. polybractea is softer and richer than *E. globulus.*

E. citriodora yields a delicate lemony scent that adds freshness to blends. *E. citriodora* is also sedating and anti-inflammatory and has a strong antiviral action. It supports recuperation from long illness.

E. globulus var. *gommier rouge* is a variety of *E. globulus* that is grown on the island of Corsica. *Gommier rouge* is the sweetest and most elegant of all the eucalyptus oils.

ROSEMARY (*Rosmarinus officinalis,* 'camphor,' 'cineol')

Rosemary oil is obtained from the fresh stalks, leaves, and flowers of the plant. The fragrance is clear, strong, and stimulating, and is easily absorbed through the skin. It is an antioxidant. It stimulates the mind, body, adrenals, and memory. Rosemary treats general weakness, mental fatigue, and sore muscles, and is used for hair and skin care.

Caution: Rosemary oil is not to be used during pregnancy. Rosemary oil should not be used internally for extended periods: A cumulative buildup can be toxic. Rosemary should be avoided by those with elevated blood pressure and anyone subject to seizures.

Therapeutic Uses

Rosemary oil is helpful for all diseases that result from a reduction of the functions of the nervous system. A strong stimulant, it clears the mind if there is confusion or doubt.

Rosemary is a tonic for the heart, liver, and gallbladder. It increases the secretion of bile and helps lower blood cholesterol. Rosemary stimulates and regulates menstruation, enhances circulation, and relieves involuntary muscle spasms.

Oil of rosemary has traditionally been used for conditioning the scalp and stimulating healthy hair growth. The pure essence, blended with lavender oil, makes a fragrant hair conditioner. I put a few drops on the top of my head before showering to help me wake up. I also put rosemary oil in a diffuser, and set the diffuser on a timer to wake me up in the morning. It is wonderful to be awakened by the invigorating scent of rosemary instead of the annoying ring of an alarm.

A few drops of rosemary oil taken with water is good for all liver and gallbladder ailments. It increases the secretion of bile and decreases blood sugar levels. It also discourages the buildup of acids in the joints that lead to arthritis.

OTHER TYPES OF ROSEMARY OIL

R. officinalis 'verbenon' is a rosemary chemotype (a composition of the essential oil in which one chemical dominates) that acts as a nervous system regulator. It also treats liver and gallbladder disorders and dry skin.

R. officinalis 'borneol' is a chemotype closer in nature to *R. officinalis.* It is used for heart and pulmonary problems, and all other rosemary applications.

R. officinalis 'Pyramidalis' is the newest chemotype.

LEMON *(Citrus limon)*

Lemon oil, derived from the peel of the lemon, has a fresh, clean scent that activates the body, dispelling sluggishness and stimulating the central nervous system.

Therapeutic Uses

Lemon's bactericidal and antiseptic properties recommend its use against infectious diseases. In Spain and other southern European countries, lemon oil is commonly used for detoxification and purification, and as a remedy for almost any ailment. It treats wrinkles, brown spots and oily skin, sore throat, dry brittle fingernails, and infectious disease.

A few drops of lemon oil, dispersed in olive oil or honey and taken with water or tea, counteracts stomach acidity and speeds up slow digestive systems. It stimulates secretions from the stomach, liver, and pancreas. Lemon oil supports the action and generation of white blood cells. Recent research in France indicates that limonene (a primary constituent of lemon oil) may be effective in the prevention of breast and other types of cancer.

CYPRESS *(Cupressus sempervirens)*

Cypress oil is obtained from the green branches, leaves, and nuts of the cypress. The oil is clear with a spicy-sweet, woodsy scent, rather masculine in character. A cypress oil bath is relaxing and refreshing.

Therapeutic Uses

Cypress oil is therapeutically indicated when heavy losses of liquid weaken the body. It is interesting to note Nicholas Culpeper's description of cypress, written in the early 17th century. Culpeper, a famous astrologer-physician, wrote, "The cones or nuts are mostly used . . . they are accounted very drying and binding, good to stop fluxes of all kinds, spitting blood, diarrhea, dysentery, the immoderate flux of the menses, involuntary micturition, they prevent the bleeding of the gums and fasten loose teeth. . . ." Although Culpeper's description may not sound very scientific in the 20th century, it remains an exact description of the oil's effect. The ability of cypress oil to halt the pathologic flow of body juices is unique. Although nothing but time will cure a fully developed flu virus, cypress oil helps tame it in its early stages. A drop of cypress oil on the pillow has an antispasmodic effect and will ease coughs.

The astringent (drying) effect of cypress oil in combination with hyssop oil can ease the suffering of hay fever. Two drops of cypress and hyssop oil taken with water in the morning, and later (if eyes begin to itch or swell) 2 drops rubbed onto the palms of the hands, provides symptomatic relief, and may result in a decrease of allergic sensitivity.

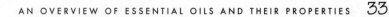

A SUPPORTIVE OIL
Cypress is excellent for smoothing transitions, particularly the loss of friends and loved ones or the ending of relationships. Inhale the fragrance for strength and comfort.

PEPPERMINT *(Mentha x piperita)*

Peppermint oil is distilled from the fresh leaves of the small, hardy perennial peppermint. The American states of Oregon, Washington, Montana, and Indiana are major producers of peppermint oil. Peppermint is also grown commercially in Germany and France.

Peppermint flavor is well known in all sorts of commercial products: chewing gums, candies, toothpaste, mouthwash, liquors. Place a drop of peppermint oil on your tongue and suck in some air to experience the distinct cooling action of menthol, the primary chemical constituent of peppermint oil. Menthol, in its chemically isolated form, is used in many pharmaceutical preparations to treat sore muscles, aches, and pains.

Peppermint oil is analgesic, antiseptic, sedative, and cooling. Children love the smell. Inhaling the scent halts negative thoughts.

Therapeutic Uses

Peppermint oil is a digestive aid, an antidepressant, an antiseptic, and an analgesic (relieves pain). It is used to treat fevers, colds, flu, nausea, respiratory disorders, and kidney and gallstones. It can help clear the sinuses, soothe a headache, and ease the misery of motion sickness. Peppermint oil is hepatic (detoxifies the liver), and an effective treatment for gaseous indigestion and irritated colon. The odorous intestinal gas resulting from the successful treatment of candida or intestinal parasites can be mitigated with peppermint.

A drop of peppermint, dissolved into a teaspoon of honey or dispersed in a teaspoon of apple cider vinegar, then taken with 8 ounces (235 ml) of fresh water, will quickly alleviate most gas and nausea.

Two drops of peppermint oil mixed into bathwater effectively cools a fever. A few drops dispersed in water and used as a compress or spray will soothe the itch and sting of insect bites.

OTHER ESSENTIAL OILS TO KNOW

The variety of essential oils available in the worldwide marketplace is constantly growing and changing. Prices and availability are affected by economics and politics, as well as weather conditions and natural disasters. The sources of essential oils are limited only by the variety of resources Mother Nature has provided. Nontraditional materials are subjected to extraction processes, and the resulting products are continually introduced to the world market. Traditional materials processed in nontraditional ways produce oils with different characteristics. As scientific research verifies traditionally accepted properties, previously unknown constituents and actions are also revealed. All of these factors contribute to a volatile world market. Therefore, the following list of essential oils, and their properties and uses, is by no means all-inclusive.

ALLSPICE (*Pimenta dioica*)

The oil is obtained from the berries of a West Indian tree of the myrtle family. Allspice is stimulating and vitalizing, and supports determination. It treats depression, nervous exhaustion, arthritis, fatigue, stiffness, flatulence, and indigestion.

AMBER (*Liquidambar orientalis* aka *Levant storax*)

Liquid amber is obtained through distillation of ambar resin, purified through redistillation. The oil has a deep, rich, smoky scent. It contains terpenes and resins. Frequently oils identified as "amber" are actually a blend of labdanum and styrax. Ambers are used in perfumery and in rituals to support the heart chakra (one of the seven body centers considered to be the source of spiritual energy).

AMBRETTE (*Abelmoschus moschatus*)

Ambrette is a vegetable "musk" produced from the musk mallow seedpod. It acts as an adrenal stimulant. Ambrette is used in perfumery and psychological work.

AMMI (*Ammi visnaga*)

Ammi oil supports respiration, and treats acute asthma. It also acts as a coronary diluent and a diuretic.

ANGELICA (*Angelica archangelica*)

Angelica is said to be the legendary scent of ageless angels. It is used in perfumery, for anorexia, and for stomach ulcers. Apply 1 drop above each breast to support the lung and heart chakras (two of the seven body centers considered to be the sources of spiritual energy).

ANISE (*Pimpinella anisum*)

Anise is a gland stimulant, and treats migraine, indigestion, irregular heartbeat, asthma, colic, impotence, and painful periods. Anise is the flavor of licorice, and the base of pastis and ouzo digestive liquors.

ARTEMIS, BLUE (*Artemisia arborescens*)

Artemis is an anti-inflammatory, mucolytic, antiallergenic, and antihistamine. It treats bronchitis, skin infections, rashes, burns, cancerous skin, and other forms of dermatitis. Blue artemis is high in azulene, a very rare, extremely soothing, powerful healing agent.

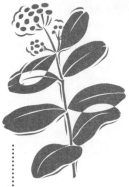

CAUTION

Angelica oil should not be used on skin prior to exposure to the sun or to tanning lights.

ASPIC *(Lavandula latifolia)*

Aspic is also known as spike lavender, a variety of lavender often used as an antiseptic in skin care. Named for the serpent (in Spanish, *spica*) whose venomous bite the plant was used to treat, aspic was also used to treat scorpion and black widow bites. Aspic was crossed with true lavender *(L. angustifolia)* to create the high-yield hybrid lavandin *(L.* x *intermedia)*.

BASIL *(Ocimum basilicum)*

Basil is used as a bath and hair oil. It treats mental stress, intellectual overwork, depression, brain damage, and memory loss and is used to forestall outbreaks of herpes and shingles. Basil can help slow down and relax the minds of children with attention deficit disorder (ADD). Place 1 drop on the child's palms, have him rub his palms briskly together, then cup them around his nose and mouth, and inhale.

BAY RUM *(Pimenta racemosa)*

Derived from the pimento berry, bay is the scent of Old Spice, the quintessential men's cologne. It treats scalp conditions, dandruff, greasy hair, muscular neuralgia, sprains, poor circulation, colds, flus, and infectious disease.

BAY LAUREL *(Laurus nobilis)*

Bay laurel has a stimulating, uplifting, somewhat masculine scent. It treats sinus headache and travel fatigue. It restores the adrenals and the immune system. Bay laurel is also an effective insect repellent.

BENZOIN *(Styrax benzoin)*

Benzoin has a warm balsamic scent. It is used as a fixative in herbal medicines and perfumes. The scent has a euphoric, sensual, and seductive quality. Benzoin is uplifting for fatigued minds. Used as an inhalation, benzoin relieves coughs and lung congestion.

BERGAMOT *(Citrus bergamia)*

Bergamot is a major component in classic Eau de Colognes and Earl Grey teas. It is antiseptic and treats psoriasis, herpes, intestinal parasites, acne, stress, depression, nervousness, eczema, and gallstones.

CAUTION

Bergamot should not be used on the skin prior to exposure to the sun or to tanning lights.

BIRCH (*Betula* spp.)

Birch bark oil is also known as sweet birch, cherry birch, southern birch, and black birch. The oil is distilled from the leaves and bark of several birch species that grow wild throughout the eastern regions of North America. Birch is used as an astringent, a counterirritant, and an antirheumatic. It treats arthritis, sore or stiff muscles, and joint pain. Birch is a popular flavoring agent, the most common source of wintergreen flavor. Birch bud oil is distilled from the leaf buds of *B. pendula* in Germany and Denmark, and *B. pubescens* in Finland. The leaf bud oil is also healing to the skin.

BITTER ALMOND (*Prunus dulcis*)

Bitter almond is the original benzylaldehyde, the "benzene ring" molecule that pushed organic chemistry into synthetic chemistry.

BLACK PEPPER (*Piper nigrum*)

Black pepper is stimulating to the mind. It restores muscle tone and promotes healthy urinary, respiratory, and digestive systems. Black pepper is used in bath and massage oils, particularly appropriate for cold weather. It treats sexual impotence problems and frigidity.

BLUE CYPRESS (*Callitris intratropica*)

Blue cypress is a new oil from Australia with a nutty, sweet, peppery odor. The primary components of blue cypress are guaiol, eudesmols, guaienes, bulnesol, furanone, and selinens. The oil is unique for its blue color. Blue cypress shows potential as an anti-inflammatory.

BLUE TANSY (*Tanacetum annuum*)

This plant is more antiallergenic and anti-inflammatory than chamomile (*Matricaria recutita*) but less effective in treating inflammation of the stomach and intestines.

BOIS DE ROSE (*Aniba rosaeodora*)

Also called rosewood oil, bois de rose is obtained from the rosewood tree, whose wood is also used to make the finest musical instruments. Native to Central and South America, bois de rose is endangered by the continued destruction of the rain forests. It is used in perfumery, and as a substitute for rose oil. Bois de rose also treats acne and other

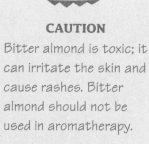

CAUTION

Bitter almond is toxic; it can irritate the skin and cause rashes. Bitter almond should not be used in aromatherapy.

CAUTION

Always dilute black pepper oil; it can be irritating to the kidneys.

skin conditions. Ten drops of bois de rose mixed with 5 drops of juniper oil and added to the bath will soothe the kidneys.

BUPLEURUM (*Bupleurum fructicosum*)

An oil new to the market, bupleurum is obtained from a wild plant in France. Bupleurum is high in limonene and A and B pinene, components valued in the French pharmaceutical industry. Bupleurum treats edema (abnormal accumulation of fluids).

CAJEPUT (*Melaleuca leucadendron* or *M. Cajuputi*)

Cajeput comes from Indonesia and Cambodia. The pungent odor of cajeput is reminiscent of eucalyptus. It treats bronchitis, laryngitis, asthma, toothache, earache, and skin diseases. The fragrance of cajeput improves mental concentration.

CAMPHOR (*Cinnamomum camphora*)

Camphor disinfects the alimentary canal and strengthens the heart. It treats infectious disease and chapped skin. Camphor has the unique dual action of cooling and heating the skin simultaneously.

CARAWAY (*Carum carvi*)

The fragrance of caraway is refreshing to the conscious mind. Sniff caraway oil to enhance alertness. Caraway acts as a stimulant and carminative, it promotes a healthy lymphatic system, and it aids circulation and digestion. Caraway treats toothache, mange in dogs, intestinal parasites, and scabies. It is also used as a flavoring agent.

CARDAMOM (*Elettaria cardamomum*)

The aroma of cardamom helps clear the conscious mind and stimulate the appetite. Cardamom acts as a digestive aid and an aphrodisiac. Its effect is felt by inhaling the fragrance. Cardamom treats colic, nausea in pregnancy, nervousness, and mental fatigue. It calms the stomach after vomiting.

CARROT SEED (*Daucus carota*)

Carrot seed oil contains vitamin A and carotene. It acts as a hepatic (detoxifies the liver) and tonic for the liver and gallbladder, and aids in retention of urine. Carrot seed oil treats aging dry skin, brown splotchy skin, blemishes, wrinkles, and skin diseases.

CAUTION

Camphor cancels out homeopathic remedies. Only use white camphor. Yellow and brown camphor are toxic.

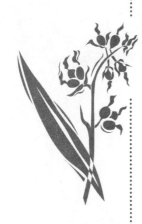

CASSIA *(Cinnamomum cassia)*

Used medicinally in much the same way as cinnamon, cassia has a warm spicy odor and acts as a carminative and antiseptic. Chinese medicine uses it for vascular disorders, but it has very few applications in aromatherapy. *Caution:* Cassia is highly irritating to the skin.

CEDARWOOD *(Cedrus atlantica)*

Cedarwood is the first oil known to have been extracted. Cedarwood acts as a sedative, astringent, and antiseptic. It treats acne, oily skin, dandruff, and other skin conditions. Cedarwood can also be used to treat respiratory and urinary infections. The scent of cedarwood promotes spirituality, balance, and calmness.

CELERY SEED *(Apium graveolens)*

Celery seed oil acts as a carminative, nerve tonic, sedative, antipigmentary (prevents skin discoloration associated with age and damage), and diuretic. It treats swollen glands, bronchitis, and congested veins. Inhale the scent to awaken psychic awareness.

CHAMOMILE *(Matricaria recutita)*

The oil of this plant, also known as blue chamomile, is a relaxing agent. Its fragrance promotes peace and reduces stress and tension. Chamomile treats inflammations of the skin, hyperallergenic conditions, hypersensitive skin, liver problems, headache, migraine, and pain elsewhere in the body. There are many varieties of blue chamomile.

CHAMOMILE, ROMAN *(Chamaemelum nobile)*

This chamomile acts as an antispasmodic, anti-inflammatory, analgesic, nerve sedative, and hepatic (liver detoxifier). It is used for skin care and treats acne, eczema, rashes, teething pain, and toothache. A few drops of Roman chamomile rubbed on the neck before a dental procedure will ease anxiety and support the anesthetic's effect.

CHAMOMILE, WILD *(Chamaemelum mixtum)*

Wild chamomile is not a true chamomile, and its effects are the opposite of those produced by the other chamomiles. It's a general stimulant.

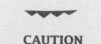

CAUTION

Cedarwood should be avoided by those with elevated blood pressure.

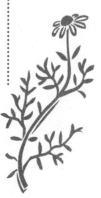

CHAMPA *(Michelia champaca)*

Champa oil is produced in India. Also known as nag champaca, it is a sweet floral absolute used in incense and perfumery. The scent promotes happiness.

CINNAMON BARK *(Cinnamomum zeylanicum)*

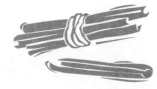

The oil obtained from cinnamon bark acts as a stimulant, an antiseptic, and an antifungal. It makes a warming bath and massage oil. The oil treats dry heaves, and is used as a sexual stimulant. The aroma of cinnamon increases your ability to tap into your psychic mind, and is reputed to increase financial prosperity. *Caution:* Cinnamon oil must be diluted. It can cause skin irritation.

CISTUS *(Cistus ladanifer)*

Cistus is a musky-scented oil obtained from the redistillation of the leaves of the rockrose. (*See* Amber and Labdanum.) It is used in perfumery. Cistus is an effective hemostatic (heals wounds, stops bleeding). It acts as a tonic for mature skin and treats wrinkles, cancer, and other skin conditions, as well as respiratory disorders, bronchitis, coughs, nervousness, and insomnia.

CITRONELLA *(Cymbopogon nardus)*

Citronella is used in perfumery and as an inexpensive scenting agent in many commercial products. It acts as a deodorant, an insect repellent, and a heart stimulant. Citronella has antiviral properties, and can be used as an ingredient in hair and massage oils. *Caution:* Citronella must be diluted. It can cause skin irritation.

CLARY SAGE *(Salvia sclarea)*

Clary has a soft, sweet, herbaceous scent. The oil is used in perfumery. Clary sage is mildly intoxicating, acts as an adrenal stimulant, and is strengthening to the stomach and kidneys. Clary is inhaled to induce euphoria, reduce emotional stress, and relieve premenstrual tension. It is also used to encourage labor and aid in childbirth.

CLOVE *(Syzygium aromaticum)*
Clove oil is extracted from the buds, leaves, and stems of an evergreen
tree native to Indonesia. The oil is used worldwide as a flavoring and
scent ingredient in food and drink, as well as toothpaste, soaps, and
cosmetics. The milder bud oil is favored for aromatherapy use. It
treats arthritis, toothache, asthma, and bronchitis. Clove oil acts as an
antibiotic, antihistamine, antioxidant, aphrodisiac, and expectorant.
Caution: Clove oil must be diluted. It can cause skin irritation.

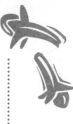

CUMIN *(Cuminum cyminum)*
Cumin is a stimulating spice in Indian and Mexican cuisine. The oil
is also used as a spice note in perfumery. As an ingredient in massage oil, it improves poor circulation. Traditionally, cumin has been
utilized for internal and home protection.

DILL WEED *(Anethum graveolens)*
Dill weed is a carminative (soothing to the stomach). The oil is useful
for treating colic in babies, and counteracting dry heaves. The oil is
also used as a flavoring agent. Sniff dill to clear the conscious mind
and sharpen awareness.

ELEMI *(Canarium luzonicum)*
Elemi oil is colorless to pale yellow with a light, fresh, balsamic-
spicy, lemonlike scent. Elemi has fortifying and regulating effects. It
acts as an antiseptic, expectorant, stimulant, and tonic.

EVERLASTING *(Helichrysum angustifolium)*
Everlasting is an anticoagulant, anti-inflammatory, and hepatocellu-
lar stimulant. It treats hematomas, bruises, contusions, phlebitis,
arthritis, hepatitis, bronchitis, spasmodic coughs, whooping cough,
tuberculosis, shingles, herpes, and acne.

FENNEL *(Foeniculum vulgare)*
Fennel is used as an aperitif (appetite stimulant) and a tonic, diuretic,
expectorant, laxative, flu preventive, and antidote for poisonous
mushrooms. It treats alcohol withdrawal and colic in babies. Fennel
stimulates estrogen and breast-milk production. Inhaling the fragrance is reputed to increase life span and instill courage.

FIR, DOUGLAS (*Pseudotsuga menziesii*)

Douglas fir treats all respiratory problems, bronchitis, urinary tract infections, and stomach cramps. It supports a healthy nervous system, and has an elevating and stabilizing effect on the mind and emotions.

FORAHA (*Calophyllum inophyllum*)

Foraha is a cold-pressed vegetable oil, included in this list for its powerful effects treating rheumatic pain, shingles, burns, rashes, impetigo, insect bites, and abrasions. It's also used topically to eliminate waste material and toxins from the capillaries, help support cellular immunity, strengthen connective tissue, and stimulate hair growth.

FRANKINCENSE (*Boswellia* spp.)

Frankincense acts as an antiseptic, expectorant, astringent (to uterine and mucous membranes), and digestive aid. It treats anxiety, nervous tension, infections of the urinary tract, leprosy, wounds, and hemorrhages. Frankincense is burned in the Catholic Church to protect against evil spirits. The scent has an elevating, warming, and soothing effect on the mind and emotions. Frankincense is ideal for meditation, because it slows and deepens the breath.

GALBANUM (*Ferula gumosa*)

Galbanum oil has a very bitter green scent that blends well with sweet florals. It is used in perfumery, and as a powerful ingredient in preparations for rejuvenating aging skin, and healing wounds and acne. Galbanum was used in ancient Egypt for embalming and incense.

GENET (*Spartium junceum*)

Genet is also known as Spanish broom. The oil has a very sweet, narcotic, honeylike fragrance. It is used in perfumery.

GINGER (*Zingiber officinale*)

Ginger oil acts as an antiseptic, laxative, tonic, stomachic (digestive tonic), and appetite stimulant. As a massage oil, it treats rheumatic pains and breaks up congested areas. Ginger can be used to provide a temporary storehouse of extra energy when needed. It is used for purification and promoting courage, confidence, aggression, and success.

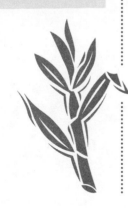

CAUTION

Genet can be toxic, and has no application in aromatherapy.

GRAPEFRUIT *(Citrus x paradisi)*

Grapefruit is an astringent and a digestive aid. It acts as a lymphatic (stimulates the lymphatic system and gallbladder). Grapefruit is used to treat obesity, cellulite, and water retention. It is also used as a facial toner and an ingredient in massage oil. The scent of grapefruit oil induces euphoria and relieves performance anxiety.

HINA *(Lawsonia inermis)*

A red oil obtained from henna, the tropical shrub that produces henna dye, hina is used in hair coloring and by East Indian women to decorate their hands, feet, and foreheads.

HONEY (from *Apis mellifera*)

Honey is a new top note used in perfumery. Warm and sweet, the scent is very soothing for children.

HYSSOP *(Hyssopus officinalis)*

Hyssop treats hay fever, asthma, coughs, hypotension, cancerous growths, eczema, sore throats, and parasites. It stimulates the medulla oblongata, and helps clear the head and vision. The scent of hyssop can heighten spirituality prior to religious rituals.

JASMINE *(Jasminum officinale)*

The fragrance of jasmine is very soothing and can be used as an aphrodisiac in love rituals. Jasmine dispels depression, is relaxing, and supports childbirth. The unique fragrance is capable of leading us into brighter worlds of fantasy and sensuality.

JUNIPER *(Juniperus communis)*

Juniper acts as an antiseptic, astringent, and diuretic. It treats diabetes, cystitis, paralysis, and arthritis. Juniper baths are invigorating, and specific for depleted kidney and bladder energy. Inhale juniper oil while visualizing protection from negativity and danger.

KEWDA *(Pandanus odoratissimus)*

Kewda is an Indian oil with a spicy-floral scent reminiscent of gardenias and horseradish. In Ayurveda (traditional Hindu medicine), kewda is used for skin care and spleen and liver support.

CAUTION

Hyssop should not be used internally for extended periods, because a cumulative buildup can be toxic. It should be avoided by those with elevated blood pressure. It is not to be used by anyone subject to seizures.

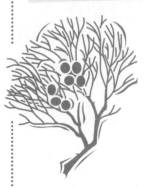

LABDANUM *(Cistus ladanifer)*

Labdanum is a floral musk derived from the leaves of the rockrose. It's used in perfumery and meditation, and to produce amber-type oils. Labdanum acts as a sedative, and treats insomnia, nervousness, and wounds. In a massage oil, it's good for spinal degeneration. (*See* Cistus.)

LEMON VERBENA *(Aloysia triphylla)*

Lemon verbena is grown commercially in Brazil and Morocco. The oil has an elegant, refreshing, and uplifting lemon scent. It is used in perfumery and skin care. Lemon verbena acts as a sedative and purifier. It treats fever, hangovers, and nervous indigestion. Lemon verbena has traditionally been used to excite spiritual love.

LEMONGRASS *(Cymbopogon citratus)*

Lemongrass has an uplifting scent. The oil is used in perfumery, and bath and massage oils. It acts as a deodorant and a purifier for oily skin. Lemongrass has antiviral, antifungal, and sedative properties. The scent of lemongrass stimulates psychic awareness and, when used with myrrh, promotes growth and change. *Caution:* Lemongrass must be diluted. It can cause skin irritation.

LIME *(Citrus aurantifolia)*

Lime oil, which has properties similar to lemon, acts as an astringent, a deodorant, and a restorative for the nervous system. It treats liver pain, bronchitis, and stomach cramps.

LINDEN BLOSSOM *(Tilia x vulgaris)*

The oil of linden blossom has a beautiful, honeylike fragrance and is used in perfumery. It acts as a nervine and a tonic, and it promotes perspiration. Good for headaches, colds, anxiety, and hysteria, it has a quieting and soothing effect in a perfume or massage oil blend.

LITSEA CUBEBA *(Litsea cubeba)*

Litsea cubeba is a lemon-scented flavoring agent, sometimes called May Chang. The oil is high in citral, similar to vervain. It treats stress, arrhythmia, high blood pressure, gas, indigestion, acne, dermatitis, and oily skin. *Caution:* Litsea cubeba is slightly toxic and causes sensitivity in some people, so do a patch test before using.

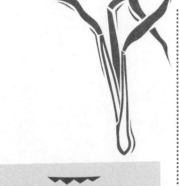

CAUTION

Lime oil should not be used on the skin prior to exposure to the sun or to tanning lights.

MACE (*Myristica fragrans*)

Mace is derived from the outer covering of the nutmeg. The oil is used in perfumery and to scent soaps. It acts as a carminative. Some people use mace as an inhalant to enhance psychic awareness.

MANDARIN (*Citrus reticulata*)

Mandarin is a very soothing oil obtained from both the green and orange fruits. Its properties resemble those of chamomile more than other citrus oils. Mandarin is very gentle and appropriate for treating indigestion, skin disorders, insomnia, restlessness, and nervous tension in pregnant women, small children, and the elderly.

MARJORAM, WILD (*Origanum vulgare*); MARJORAM, SWEET (*O. majorana*)

Marjoram is a powerful sedative. It treats insomnia, arthritis, asthma, colds, colic, migraine, nervous tension, muscle spasms, rheumatic pain, sprains, bruises, and excessive sexuality. Marjoram is useful in allaying anxiety, grief, and love obsession, as well as supporting celibacy. Sweet marjoram is also called the true garden marjoram.

MASTIC (*Pistacia lentiscus*)

Mastic is a resin with antiseptic, anti-inflammatory properties. It is used in perfumery as a warm bass note. Mastic is also a chief ingredient in a classic Greek confection.

MELISSA (*Melissa officinalis*)

Melissa acts as a general tonic and rejuvenator. It treats allergies, depression, fever, indigestion, nausea, vertigo, shock, nervous tension, menstrual irregularities, and infertility. Extensive German research has found it valuable as a topical treatment for herpes. Inhale the fragrance to lessen grief from the loss of a spouse or partner. Melissa supports peace of mind and emotional serenity, especially for women.

MIMOSA (*Acacia* spp.)

Mimosa oil is used in perfumery and for general skin care. It treats oily skin, anxiety, stress, and oversensitivity. Mimosa can be used with visualization to bring love. Anointing the forehead with a drop of mimosa before retiring will stimulate prophetic dreams.

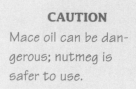

CAUTION

Mace oil can be dangerous; nutmeg is safer to use.

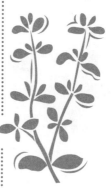

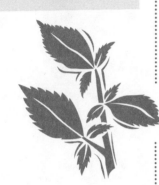

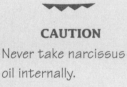

MQV (*Melaleuca viridiflora* var. *rubriflora*)

MQV acts as an antiseptic, an antibiotic, and an analgesic. It treats flu virus, urinary infections, and respiratory ailments. In France MQV, called *gomenol,* is used in place of antibiotics. (*See also* Niaouli.)

MUGWORT (*Artemisia vulgaris*)

Oil of mugwort is calming and regulating for the the female cycle. It treats sinusitis, nervousness, depression, bipolar disorder, sore muscles, colds, bronchitis, poison oak, and genital warts. Mugwort herb is used in moxibustion, part of some acupuncture treatments.

MYRRH (*Commiphora myrrha*)

The ancient Egyptians used myrrh for embalming. It is cooling to the skin, anti-inflammatory, antifungal, and purifying. It treats uterine disorders, laryngitis, cuts, cracked heels, wounds, ulcers, and wasting degenerative disease. Myrrh can enhance visualization, expand awareness, and calm fears about the future.

MYRTLE, GREEN (*Myrtus communis*)

Green myrtle is used as an ingredient in antiseptic skin washes and douches, as a treatment for diarrhea, as a tonic for the respiratory system, and as an energy system balancer. Myrtle is a traditional emblem of love.

NARCISSUS (*Narcissus poeticus*)

Narcissus oil has a sweet floral scent, with a mild narcotic effect. It is soothing to the nerves and relaxing to the mind. The lovely fragrance has long been used to manifest new relationships, or to enrich love that is already shared with another.

NEROLI (*Citrus aurantium*)

Neroli is the heady, rich scent of orange blossom. The oil acts as a sedative and a skin softener. It treats insomnia, nervous skin rashes, and stretch marks. Neroli is used in perfumery. The fragrance is light and refreshing, joyous and uplifting.

NIAOULI (*Melaleuca viridiflora* var. *rubriflora*)

Niaouli is antiseptic and protects the immune system from viruses. It treats infections, influenza, laryngitis, bronchitis, earache, wounds, and burns. To combat a psychic attack from another, inhale and visualize the niaouli energy mixing with yours, forming a barrier against negative energy. (*See also* MQV.)

NIGHT QUEEN *(Cestrum nocturnum)*
A night-scented tuberoselike flower. The oil, used in perfumery, has a narcotic quality.

NUTMEG *(Myristica fragrans)*
Nutmeg is a strong psychostimulant, carminative, and digestive stimulant. It treats rheumatism and diarrhea. Inhaling the fragrance of nutmeg opens the conscious mind to attract financial prosperity.

OAKMOSS *(Evernia prunastri)*
The scent of oakmoss is the sweet earthy scent of forest lichen. It is used in perfumery as an earthy bass note for chypre blends (see page 152). It treats headache and congested sinuses. Oakmoss can be used in visualization to increase personal and financial prosperity.

OPOPANAX *(Commiphora erythrea)*
The musty balsamic smell of opopanax is used in perfumery. The oil is antiseptic, antispasmodic, and expectorant. The applications of opopanax in aromatherapy are similar to those of myrrh.

ORANGE *(Citrus sinensis)*
Orange oil is derived from sweet orange peel. It is used in baths and skin care to revive wrinkled skin. Orange oil is calming, antigenic (produces antibodies), and humectant (plumps up dry skin). It treats nervous anxiety and intestinal gas. The fragrance of orange promotes happiness.

OREGANO *(Origanum vulgare)*
Oregano acts as a stimulant, an antiseptic, an expectorant, an analgesic, and a muscle relaxant. Oregano has recently been found to lower blood lipid levels. It is also useful for energizing you to accomplish household tasks. *Caution:* Oregano must be diluted. It can be irritating to the skin.

CAUTION

Nutmeg is toxic in large doses. Do not add nutmeg oil to bathwater. Always dilute before applying to the skin.

OSMANTHUS (Osmanthus fragrans)

Osmanthus is a tiny Chinese flower with a scent like neroli and jasmine. The oil is used in perfumery.

ORRISROOT (Iris pallida)

Orrisroot is the bulb of the iris. It is used in perfumery and extensively in European cosmetics, dentifrices, toothpastes, and diuretics. It treats colic, hoarseness, and coughs. Orris is also used in love rituals; spread it on bedsheets to induce amorous feelings.

PALMAROSA (Cymbopogon martinii)

Palmarosa is a lemony, rose-scented grass from the Philippines. The oil is hydrating and refreshing. It is used in perfumery and skin care. Palmarosa treats wrinkles and acne, and acts as a cellular stimulant. It is used in love-attracting rituals.

PARSLEY (Petroselinum crispum)

Parsley benefits nerve centers in the head and spine. It is a diuretic, and soothing to the stomach, kidneys, spleen, and intestines. Parsley treats aging skin, cellulite, and menopausal symptoms.

PATCHOULI (Pogostemon cablin)

Patchouli oil has been used for centuries in India to scent clothing and bodies. It acts as a sedative and nerve stimulant. Patchouli supports the endocrine system, and treats edema, obesity, loose sagging skin, anxiety, and depression. Considered to be rejuvenating, the scent induces peace of mind, integrates energy, and keeps us in touch with our physical selves. It awakens in us the desire to transcend boundaries and enter a state of total union with our beloved.

PENNYROYAL (Mentha pulegium)

Pennyroyal oil acts as liver and spleen tonic and a flea repellent. It treats motion sickness, nervous disturbances, toothache, headache, fever, and female disorders. Pennyroyal is used in protection rituals.

PERU BALSAM (Myroxylon balsamum var. pereirae)

Used in perfumery, Peru balsam acts as a stimulant, an expectorant, a disinfectant, and a stomachic (digestive tonic). It treats skin sores, ringworm, and stomach ulcers.

CAUTION

Pennyroyal is an abortive. It is not to be used during pregnancy.

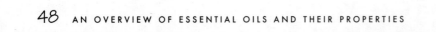

PETITGRAIN (*Citrus aurantium*)

Petitgrain is obtained from the leaves of the orange tree. The oil, used in perfumery, has a fresh, invigorating, bitter-floral fragrance. It acts as a tonic, antiseptic, antispasmodic, and digestive aid. Petitgrain sharpens awareness.

PINE (*Pinus* spp.)

Pine is antiseptic for the respiratory tract and it treats pneumonia, asthma, and other respiratory ailments. It also treats fatigue, flu, gout, joint pain, and kidney and bladder ailments. Pine acts as a male stimulant and restorative. It stimulates the adrenal cortex, which is responsible for producing steroidal (sex) hormones. Pine is added to massage and bath oils. It is also used magically for protection and attracting money.

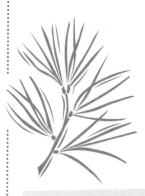

RAVENSARA (*Ravensara aromatica*)

The scent of ravensara oil resembles that of eucalyptus and cloves. Ravensara has antibacterial, antiviral, and immuno-modulating properties. It treats chicken pox and shingles (herpes zoster).

ROSE GERANIUM (*Pelargonium graveolens*)

Rose geranium oil is used in perfumery, massage oils, and potpourris. It has the same rejuvenating properties as geranium. It calms and refreshes the psyche and body. (*See* Zdravetz, a new oil from Bulgaria derived from wild geranium.)

ROSE (*Rosa gallica*); ROSE, BULGARIAN (*R. x damascena*); ROSE, EGYPTIAN (*R. x centifolia*); ROSE, MOROC (*R. x centifolia*); ROSE, TURKEY (*R. multiflora*)

Each rose oil has a unique scent. Bulgarian is the finest. All of the rose oils are used in perfumery. They are cooling and soothing to sensitive skin. Rose oil supports a healthy liver, stomach, and blood. It increases semen in men, and is cleansing and regulating for the female sexual organs. Rose acts as a laxative tonic for psychological impotence. It treats depression and melancholy, and calms domestic strife. The fragrance of the rose has the power to unite physical and spiritual love, the source of beauty, joy, and happiness.

CAUTION

Ravensara aromatica should not be confused with *Ravensara anisata*, which is abortive in excessive doses and should not to be used during pregnancy or by asthmatics.

RUE (*Ruta graveolens*)

Rue has been used as a magical herb by many cultures.

SAGE (*Salvia officinalis*)

Sage acts as a nerve and adrenal stimulant. It restores energy to the whole organism. The oil is used in the bath, to relieve labor pains and the discomforts of menopause, and to dry up breast milk. Sage incites wisdom.

ST.-JOHN'S-WORT (*Hypericum perforatum*)

St.-John's-wort is a hardy perennial that produces a profusion of fragrant lemony-scented flowers. The oil is an astringent, and treats cuts and burns. It balances the chakras (seven body centers considered to be the sources of spiritual energy), and treats depression and nerve and spinal trauma, especially whiplash injuries. St.-John's-wort heals emotional pain when you are very sensitive.

SANDALWOOD (*Santalum album*)

Sandalwood is a sweet woody scent used in perfumery and massage oils. It treats dry skin, bladder infections, nervous tension, acne, strep and staph infections, gonorrhea, diarrhea, and depression. Sandalwood acts as a sedative and an aphrodisiac. Inhale the fragrance to instill spirituality and inner quiet.

SASSAFRAS (*Sassafras albidum*)

The oil is used in perfumery. It treats arthritis, skin disease, poison oak and ivy, and exhaustion.

SASSAFRAS, BRAZILIAN (*Ocotea cymbarum*)

This is the sassafras that produces the familiar root beer scent. The bark is used in an herb tea as a cleanser.

SAVORY (*Satureja montana*)

Savory oil, distilled from the plant commonly known as winter or mountain savory, is pale yellow to clear with a sharp, herbaceous, medicinal scent. It is used extensively in French aromatherapy for its strong antifungal action. It is also astringent and anticatarrhal, and acts as stimulant and an aphrodisiac. *Caution:* Savory must be diluted. It can be irritating to the skin.

SPEARMINT *(Mentha spicata)*

Spearmint is stimulating and refreshing to skin and muscles. It is used as an appetite stimulant. Spearmint oil treats all women's complaints. It is used in massage and bath oils, in douches, and as a flavoring agent.

SPIKENARD *(Nardostachys jatamansi)*

Spikenard was the oil Mary Magdalene used to anoint Christ. It is considered to be antiaging and is used to treat incurable skin troubles.

SPRUCE *(Picea* **spp.)**

Spruce oil, obtained from Canadian silver and white spruce trees, acts as an expectorant and a respiratory antiseptic. It treats lung congestion and tightens watery tissues.

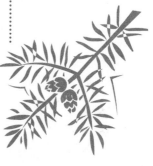

STAR ANISE *(Illicium verum)*

Star anise acts as an antiseptic, a digestive, and an expectorant. It treats colic, cramps, joint pain, rheumatism, bronchitis, coughs, and other respiratory problems. It is also an insect repellent.

STYRAX *(Liquidambar styraciflua)*

Styrax, sometimes called storax, is a semiliquid, resinous gum used in perfumery and skin care. Mixed with labdanum, it is used to make amber oil. Styrax treats ringworm, scabies, colds, coughs, and catarrh (inflammation of a mucous membrane).

TANGERINE *(Citrus reticulata)*

Tangerine oil is mild and appropriate for use on children. It supports the peripheral circulatory system and is used to treat acne, oily skin, fluid retention, stretch marks, insomnia, and nervous tension.

TARRAGON *(Artemisia dracunculus)*

Tarragon acts as an aperitif (appetite stimulant). It balances the nervous system and treats anorexia, hiccups, intestinal spasms, nervous indigestion, painful periods, and menstrual irregularities.

TEA TREE *(Melaleuca alternifolia)*

Tea trea has been used for thousands of years by the Aboriginal people of Australia. The oil is antiseptic, nonirritating, nontoxic, and an energy stimulant. It treats acne, skin rashes, fungal infections,

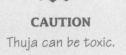
tooth and gum infections, vaginal infections, respiratory problems, immune system deficiencies, strep throat, staph, and chicken pox. Tea tree can be applied directly to the skin or taken orally.

TEREBINTH (*Pinus pinaster*)

Terebinth acts as an antiseptic and analgesic. The oil is used in baths. It loosens bronchial phlegm and supports pulmonary and genitourinary health. Terebinth treats gallstones, constipation, colitis, and parasites. The oil is obtained from various species.

THUJA CEDAR (*Thuja occidentalis*)

Also commonly called the white cedar tree, the oil from the thuja cedar acts as a diuretic and urinary sedative. It is soothing and relaxing in the bath. Thuja treats enlarged prostate, impotence, and warts.

THYME (*Thymus vulgaris*)

Thyme oil acts as general stimulant, brain stimulant, and skin antiseptic. It treats fatigue, mental exhaustion, infectious disease, sore throat, acne, respiratory disease, yeast infection, and *Candida albicans.*

CHEMOTYPES OF THYME OIL

A chemotype is chemical composition of the essential oil in which one chemical dominates.

Thymus vulgaris 'linalol' ct 3 is antiseptic. Good for sensitive skin.

Thymus vulgaris 'geraniol' is antiseptic and antifungal.

Thymus vulgaris 'thujanol' is a mild antiseptic.

Thymus vulgaris 'thymol' is also antiseptic.

TOLU BALSAM (*Myroxylon balsamum*)

Tolu acts as a stimulant, a tonic, and an expectorant. It is used in perfumery and cosmetics, and as an ingredient in cough syrups. It treats cracked nipples, eczema, rashes, wounds, and scabies. Tolu was known and used by the Aztecs.

TONKA *(Dipteryx odorata)*

Tonka produces a sweet vanilla, musky-type scent, and is used as a fixative in perfumery. Tonka is valued for its aphrodisiac and narcotic effects. It is also used as an insecticide.

TRIFOLIA *(Zanthoxylum alatum)*

Trifolia oil is obtained from the fruit of a Himalayan prickly ash. The pungent, sweet oil is used in perfumery and in Ayurveda (traditional Hindu medicine) to relieve dental pain and treat constipation, yeast infection, and parasites.

TUBEROSE *(Polianthes tuberosa)*

The narcotic scent of tuberose calms and soothes the emotions and helps you gain self-control. It invites love through visualization, and it is reputed to still raging passions.

TURMERIC *(Curcuma longa)*

Turmeric oil is obtained from the same gold-colored rhizome that produces a component of curry. Used in Chinese medicine as a digestive tonic, laxative, diuretic, hypotensive, and anti-inflammatory, turmeric treats bruises, abdominal pain, colic, and muscle and joint pain.

UD *(Agollocha aquillaria)*

Ud is also known as aloeswood, agarwood, and oud. Ud is the scent of ancient temples, magic, and ceremonies. It has been used for centuries in Asia as a funeral scent. Ud is used as perfume and incense in Arabia. Sufis believe a drop of ud placed in the ear will assist you in reaching the highest stations of the soul.

VERVAIN LIPPIA *(Aloysia triphylla)*

Vervain is used in perfumery and soaps. It acts as an expectorant and tranquilizer, and treats coughs and colds, cramps, liver congestion, insomnia, nervous stress, and oily skin. The fragrance of vervain stimulates creativity.

VETIVER *(Vetiveria zizanioides)*

Vetiver is used in perfumery and as a moisturizing bath oil. It acts as a sedative and treats insomnia. Vetiver is also an effective moth repellent. It blends well with sandalwood and rose.

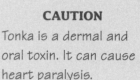

CAUTION

Tonka is a dermal and oral toxin. It can cause heart paralysis.

VIOLET LEAF *(Viola odorata)*

Violet leaf is used in perfumery and skin care. The oil acts as a sedative, a liver decongestant, and a circulatory stimulant. It treats aging and problem skin, blackheads, and enlarged pores. Violet leaf supports the emotions and heart. It soothes nostalgia and obsession.

WINTERGREEN *(Gaultheria procumbens)*

Wintergreen is an antiseptic and an analgesic. It treats sore muscles and joints and sciatica. Wintergreen blends well with juniper and *Eucalyptus citriodora.* It is a popular flavoring agent.

WORMWOOD *(Artemisia absinthium)*

Wormwood was the basis for absinthe, a popular and highly addictive French liqueur that was banned in the early 1900s. Wormwood has a very high thujone content.

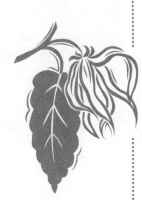

YARROW *(Achillea millefolium)*

Yarrow acts as an anti-inflammatory and supports a healthy respiratory system. It treats headaches, menstrual problems, and severe wounds and boils. Yarrow provides protection from ticks. It is also used to counter the ill effects of radiation therapy.

YLANG YLANG *(Cananga odorata)*

The voluptuous scent of ylang ylang is used in perfumery and exotic hair, bath, and body oils. The oil regulates cardiac and respiratory rhythms, and soothes anger and physical pain. It acts as an aphrodisiac, a sedative, and a euphoric. Ylang ylang treats frigidity, impotence, depression, insomnia, oily skin, acne, and insect bites. Ylang super, also called ylang extra, refers to the first press. Subsequent pressings are mixed together to make "regular" ylang. The super or extra has a superior, soft, and delicate scent.

ZDRAVETZ *(Geranium macrorrhizum)*

Zdravetz is a fairly new oil produced in Bulgaria and derived from a wild variety of geranium (a true geranium, not a pelargonium). It is used in men's perfumes. Zdravetz is a soothing oil with analgesic, antimicrobial, and antifungal properties. It also acts as an insect repellent.

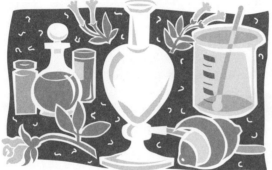

Aromachemistry

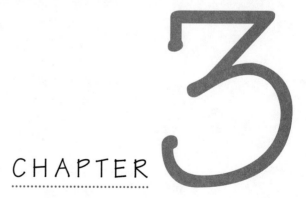

I have found that anyone interested in aromatherapy will inevitably want to learn about the chemical composition and properties of essential oils. I've always relied on my intuitive understanding of nature and its products, and had never planned to undertake a study of chemistry. But this is a very exciting time in aromatherapy. The essential oil industry is expanding rapidly, and with the explosion in popularity of aromatherapy more and more oils are being scrutinized by science. As various essential oils become the subject of increasingly penetrating research into their composition, traditionally accepted properties are confirmed, common constituents are identified, and previously unknown constituents and actions are demonstrated. Eventually I realized that it was imperative for me to have a rudimentary understanding of essential oil chemistry, which, while intimidating, actually led me to a deeper understanding of aromatherapy. I discovered that the hard, technical science of chemistry was a complement to my softer, intuitive, and spiritual understanding of aromatherapy.

BUILDING BLOCKS OF AROMA

Essential oils are compounds made up of aromatic molecules. Organic chemistry examines the compounds made up of carbon, hydrogen, nitrogen, and oxygen atoms, the bonds between carbon atoms and other carbon atoms, and the bonds between carbon atoms and hydrogen atoms. These are the basic molecular building blocks of living organisms. In the same way that we have cells, tissues, and systems in our bodies, we also have atoms, molecules, and compounds, which range from minute to visible in size.

Carbon atoms bond together in chains. These chains can be structured in a straight line, branched, or formed into a ring.

An isoprene is a branched structure composed of five carbon atoms, onto which hydrogen can easily bond. Isoprenes form the basic building blocks of aromatic molecules.

Terpenes are molecules made up of carbon and hydrogen atoms. As a circumstance of their chemical structure, terpenes — particularly monoterpenes — are vulnerable to oxidation. Indeed, oxidation is the main cause of spoilage in essential oils, such as the citrus oils, that are rich in monoterpenes.

A monoterpene is a molecule composed of two isoprene units, or 10 carbon atoms joined head to tail. Monoterpenes occur in almost all essential oils. Limonene, for example, is a monoterpene that occurs as a major constituent of lemon oil, as well as occurring in smaller quantities in many other essential oils.

Sesquiterpenes have three isoprene units, or 15 carbon atoms joined together head to tail. This makes a denser molecular structure, which causes sesquiterpenes to evaporate more slowly than monoterpenes. Sesquiterpenes are a common constituent in essential oils and make very significant contributions to their odors. The zingiberene in ginger oil is an example of a sesquiterpene.

The other basic building block for essential oil molecules is the joining of six carbon atoms in a ring structure, called a benzene (aromatic) or phenyl ring.

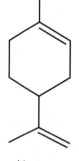

Limonene

FUNCTIONAL GROUPS

When other atoms bond to these two basic structures, we have what are called functional groups: special arrangements of atoms in a molecule that are subject to characteristic chemical behavior. The chemical behavior and effect of an essential oil can be predicted through an understanding of this chemical structure. (The chart on page 59 outlines oils in the most common functional groups.)

The composition of an essential oil from a plant of a single species always follows the same general pattern, but it will differ in detail from sample to sample. The chemicals most dominant in a particular essential oil will indicate the probable action of that oil. The activity of certain essential oils is dominated by the properties

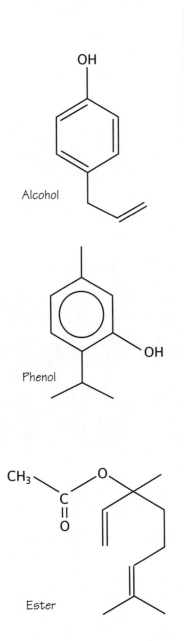

Alcohol

Phenol

Ester

of one class of chemical compounds. This may be a result of a quantitative dominance of a particular compound (or class of compound). Another possibility is that the compound has such a high level of activity that even small amounts suffice to dominate the character of the essential oil, as with lemon.

Alcohols and Phenols

Alcohols and phenols are similarly structured molecules. Both are common constituents in essential oils, but with distinctly different chemical behaviors: A phenol is highly subject to oxidation, whereas an alcohol is highly resistant to it. Thus a phenol will darken, or redden, with age. Both alcohols and phenols will form esters in reaction with organic acids.

Most alcohols that occur in essential oils possess soft, sweet, herbaceous, or woody odors. You will recognize the *ol* ending in many common constituents, such as geraniol, linalol, menthol, santol, and so on.

A phenol odor is typically medicinal in character, as with thymol, a major constituent of both thyme- and oregano-type oils, and carvacrol, a constituent that occurs widely in oils of plants from the *Labiatae* family. Phenols can also smell pungent and spicy, as does eugenol, the characteristic scent of clove. Eugenol occurs in many other oils as well, including cinnamon, rose, and ylang ylang.

Esters

Esters are the result of a chemical reaction between organic acids and alcohols or phenols, and are widely represented in essential oils. They usually provide fruity notes: Examples include the benzyl acetate in jasmine, ylang ylang, and neroli oils; the geranyl acetate in geranium, citronella, lavender, and petitgrain; and the linalyl acetate in bergamot, lavender, and clary sage.

EFFECTS OF ESSENTIAL OILS ASSOCIATED WITH FUNCTIONAL GROUPS

Functional Group	Effects of Corresponding Oils
Alcohols (monoterpenes)	Largest user-friendly group; balancing
Phenols	Aggressive antibacterials
Esters	Safest of all the essential oils; can be used "neat" (undiluted on the skin)
Aldehydes	Calming to the emotions, irritating to the skin
Ketones	Toxic, powerful, aggressive against mucus and abnormal cell growth
Ethers	Soothing to the digestive tract but will irritate in a bath
Sesquiterpenes	Most soothing and calming

Just as organic acids react with alcohols to form esters, the reverse will also occur. High-ester essential oils that contain a proportion of dissolved water from the distillation process can develop acids. The increased acidity that will develop in "moist" ester-containing oils presents an unpleasant sour smell, and is equated with spoilage.

Amines and imines are a subgroup of naturally occurring esters that lend an unpleasant note to some odors. Amines account for a sharp chemical odor in some citrus oils, as well as ylang ylang, jasmine, and tuberose. The imine indole lends a heavy animalistic note to jasmine and orange flower. Skatole, an imine highly present in civet, has more of a role in perfumery. The powerful fecal odor of skatole, when used with great discretion by a highly skilled blender, can actually add beautiful fragrance effects.

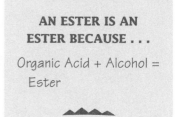

AN ESTER IS AN ESTER BECAUSE . . .

Organic Acid + Alcohol = Ester

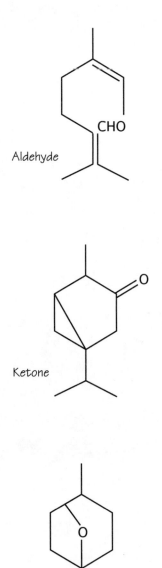

Aldehyde

Ketone

Ether

Aldehydes

Aldehydes occur in nature as minor constituents in citrus and other essential oils, as well as major constituents in a few tropical oils. Naturally occurring aldehydes include the citrals neral and geranial, found in lemon and lemongrass oils, and citronellal, found in citronella and eucalyptus oils. Aldehyde odors range from sharp and lemony through floral to intensely green. A wide range of aldehydes is manufactured synthetically for use in perfumery.

Ketones

The family of ketones exhibits a broad range of odor types. For example, methyl heptenone is a ketone occurring in lemongrass and litsea cubeba oils that gives a green, oily, rather coarse odor. Methyl amyl ketone is a minor constituent of clove oil that provides a fruity odor, and menthone is a ketone found in peppermint and other mint oils that provides a fresh, dry odor.

Note: For the purpose of consistency, the spelling *ketone* is used throughout this text. However, the spelling *cetone* (or *ceton*) is also correct, and often used in aromatherapy references.

Ethers

Ethers are relatively stable compounds, thus essential oils that are rich in ethers (such as aniseed and fennel) are particularly stable oils. Ethers contribute a variety of odors, from light and sweet to pungent and medicinal. Anethole, estragole, methyl para-cresol, and safrole are naturally occurring esters that contribute to the warm, sweet odors of licorice-like scents, including basil and tarragon.

ESSENTIAL OILS GROUPED BY CHEMICAL FAMILIES

Chemical Family	Essential Oil
Phenols	
Syzygium aromaticum	Clove
Cuminum cyminum	Cumin
Origanum vulgare	Oregano
Satureja montana	Savory
Thymus vulgaris	Thyme
Ethers	
Artemisia dracunculus	Tarragon
Ocimum basilicum	Basil
Pimpinella anisum	Aniseed
Foeniculum vulgare	Fennel
Alcohols (C_{10}) (monoterpenes)	
Aniba rosaeodora	Rosewood/Bois de Rose
Citrus aurantium	Neroli
Citrus bergamia	Bergamot
Thymus vulgaris 'linaloliferum'	Sweet Thyme
Pelargonium x asperum	Geranium
Mentha x piperita	Peppermint
Melaleuca alternifolia	Tea Tree
Melissa officinalis	Melissa
Origanum vulgare	Wild Marjoram
Origanum majorana	Sweet Marjoram
Daucus carota	Carrot Seed
Cupressus sempervirens	Cypress
Santalum album	Sandalwood

Chemical Family	Essential Oil
Oxides (1.8 Cineol) + Alcohols (C_{10})	
Eucalyptus globulus	Eucalyptus
Eucalyptus radiata	Eucalyptus radiata
Ravensara aromatica	Ravensara aromatica
Myrtus communis 'linalol'	Myrtle
Lavandula latifolia	Spike
Oxides (1.8 Cineol) + Alcohols (C_{15}) (Sesquiterpenes)	
Melaleuca viridiflora var. rubriflora	Niaouli/MQV
Oxide (1.8 Cineol) + Ester	
Laurus nobilis	Bay Laurel
Oxide (1.8 Cineol) + Ketone	
Rosmarinus officinalis 'cineol'	Rosemary
Esters	
Lavandula angustifolia ssp. angustifolia*	Lavender
Lavandula angustifolia	Miller maillette floris
Ammi visnaga	Ammi
Salvia sclarea	Clary Sage
Juniperus communis	Juniper
Cistus ladanifer	Rockrose/Cistus
Chamaemelum nobile	Roman Chamomile
Pelargonium x asperum	Geranium
Ester + Alcohols	
Cananga odorata	Ylang Ylang

(chart continued on next page)

Chemical Family	Essential Oil		Chemical Family	Essential Oil
Ester + Lacton			**Terpenes (C_{10}) Carbon + 10 bonds**	
Inula graveolens	Inula/Sweet inula		Myristica fragrans	Nutmeg
Ester + Diceton			Pinus spp.	Pine
Helichrysum angustifolium	Helichryse/Everlasting/Immortelle		Pinus spp.	Turpentine
			Citrus limon	Lemon (peel)
Aldehydes			Citrus aurantium	Orange (peel)
Aloysia triphylla	Lemon Verbena		Pistacia lentiscus	Mastic
Cymbopogon citratus	Lemongrass		**Hydrocarbons**	
Eucalyptus citriodora	Eucalyptus citriodora		Hypericum perforatum	St.-John's-Wort
Cymbopogon nardus	Citronella (Ceylon)		**Sesquiterpenes (C_{15})**	
Cymbopogon winterianus	Citronella (Java)		Apium graveolens	Celery seed
Cinnamomum zeylanicum	Cinnamon		Matricaria recutita	German Chamomile
Melissa officinalis	Melissa		Nardostachys jatamansi	Spikenard
Ketones			Achillea millefolium	Yarrow
Rosmarinus officinalis 'camphor'	Rosemary		**Sesquiterpenes (C_{15}) + Ketone**	
Rosmarinus officinalis 'verbenon'	Rosemary		Artemisia arborescens	Blue Artemis
Eucalyptus dives	Eucalyptus			
Salvia officinalis	Sage			
Cuminum cyminum	Cumin			
Hyssopus officinalis	Hyssop			
Hyssopus officinalis 'decumbens'	Hyssop			
Thuja occidentalis	Thuja cedar			

*Other species of lavenders that are not in the ester group:
   Lavandula latifolia L.F. Medikus floris
   Lavandula x intermedia
   Lavandula hybrida abrialis (10% camphor)
   Lavandula hybrida rosso
   Lavandula hybrida var. reydovan (monoterpenic alcohols)
   Lavandula stoechas (70–80% cetones)
   Lavandula hybrida super linalol does contain esters.

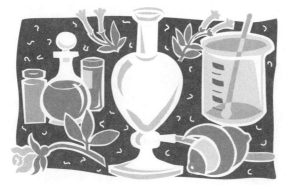

Safety
and Toxicity
Guidelines

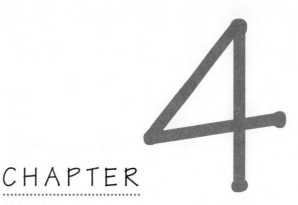

CHAPTER 4

The effective and efficient practice of aromatherapy requires education and caution. As a holistic medical therapy, aromatherapy utilizes the powerful actions of essential oils. The adage "Less is more" is one to keep in mind when working with essential oils. They are powerful, active substances that should be used in small amounts. Each drop of essential oil is filled with a host of aromatic molecules, many of which may present a certain degree of toxicity.

Before using any essential oil, you should be aware of its probable and possible effects. A great number of essential oils are benign; they do not present any toxicity when used at the correct dose. I refer to these oils as "user friendly." Some essential oils, however, are highly toxic and have no place in aromatherapy. Others have a moderate degree of toxicity and need to be used with caution. Some essential oils present a danger only after prolonged use. The best safety practice in aromatherapy is to arm yourself with reliable information.

It is important to note that essential oils are able to cross the placental barrier. They are also present in a mother's milk. Therefore, if you are pregnant or nursing, be aware that any aromatherapy treatment you undergo will affect your baby equally. You would be well advised, during this period of your life, to forgo any aromatherapy treatment that incorporates powerful oils that are to be used with caution.

Correct dosage will vary with the individual, and is determined after careful consideration of such variables as body size, weight, age, and state of health.

TOXICITY

There are different types of toxicity that need to be recognized when working with essential oils.

♦ Acute toxicity manifests within minutes after the introduction of an essential oil into the organism.

- Short-term toxicity may take from 3 to 12 months to manifest.
- Long-term toxicity can manifest after one to several years of use, as with the cumulative effect of ketones.
- Allergic reactions are the result of an individual's unique immune system response to an essential oil each time it is presented. A "specific allergic reaction" is an isolated allergic response that is not repeated upon subsequent exposures.

The two chemical groups that present the highest risk of toxicity are the ketones and the phenols.

Dangerous Ketones

Ketones can be deadly. Although they don't cause pain or burn the skin, as little as 8 to 10 drops of a high-ketone essential oil can kill a small child. Essential oils that are high in ketones can cause liver or neurotoxicity and must be used with extreme caution.

The value of high-ketone essential oils lies both in their powerful lytic (dissolving) action and in their ability to support the regeneration of injured tissue, but they should never be administered, either internally or externally, in doses higher than 6 drops per day. Although effective doses vary with the individual, an average dose is 1 to 3 drops per day. More than this can cause depression, epileptic seizures, and even death.

It is important to realize that ketones have a cumulative effect. For example, consider that the normal person can metabolize 5 drops of a high-ketone essential oil every 24 hours. If that person is dosing at 6 drops per day, on the second day she is receiving an effective dose of 7 drops. Project forward and you can see that by the 10th day, the dose is at a dangerous level. These are powerful essential oils that should be used with extreme caution.

Oils with high ketone content include rosemary, thuja, hyssop, mugwort, and cumin.

HAZARDOUS OILS

Some essential oils that are valued for their powerful action are also considered hazardous. Such oils are to be used only in very small doses and with extreme caution. If you aren't absolutely sure of all of the probable and possible actions of the following essential oils, don't use them.

- Cinnamon leaf
- Cassia
- Pennyroyal
- Thuja
- Mugwort

Dangerous Phenols

Essential oils with a high phenol content have very powerful antiseptic, antiviral, and antifungal actions, but they can burn the skin and mucous membranes, and can be toxic to the liver. It is always necessary to dilute high-phenol essential oils. Never use more than a 3 percent solution. Essential oils with high phenol content should not be diffused into the atmosphere. Phenols should never be administered to young children, or to anyone who has had viral hepatitis or a compromised liver of any sort. When essential oils rich in phenols are utilized, they are administered in an antibiotic fashion: A specific dose is given for a maximum of 10 to 12 days, just long enough to eliminate the targeted infection.

Essential oils with high phenol content include thyme, oregano, savory, clove, caraway, cinnamon, and bay (pimenta berry).

SKIN SENSITIZERS

Some essential oils are known as skin sensitizers, for their ability to increase the affectability of the skin. This can be desirable — for instance, a skin sensitizer might enhance the action of another essential oil — but can also cause redness and generalized sensitivity. The severity of the reaction may increase with subsequent exposure. Sensitivity can show as redness, itchy skin, blisters, or welts.

Oils with a probable or possible sensitizing action include benzoin, bay laurel, basil, fennel, citronella, litsea cubeba, Peru balsam, Tolu balsam, turpentine, ginger, lemongrass, and ylang ylang.

Photosensitizers

Some essential oils can cause your skin to become especially sensitive to the ultraviolet rays emitted by direct sunlight, sunlamps, and tanning beds. These oils should never be used before exposure

---

▼▼▼

BLOOD PRESSURE ELEVATORS

Some essential oils are known to raise blood pressure. Therefore, anyone with high blood pressure or considered at risk for heart attack or stroke should not use:

- Rosemary
- Cedarwood
- Hyssop
- Sage
- Thyme (common)

▲▲▲

to such light. Doing so can cause severe sunburn or permanent skin pigmentation (red blotches), and may even lead to the development of skin cancers.

Essential oils with known photosensitizing properties are bergamot, lemon, orange, lemon verbena, cumin, angelica, and lime.

Skin Irritants

Essential oils known as skin irritants can cause a rash, itchiness, or irritation that may last from 20 minutes to an hour. Also known as counterirritants, these essential oils stimulate circulation and provoke a release of endorphins that can be effective in reducing pain. In small amounts, their effect can be positive. In large doses, they can cause increased pain and inflammation and even damage to the skin. Cells may be destroyed and scarring may result.

Essential oils that are classified as counterirritants include allspice, anise, basil, black pepper, cedar (Virginia), peppermint, thyme (common), eucalyptus, caraway, and cajeput.

BATHING PRECAUTIONS

The addition of a few drops of the right essential oil can do more to enhance your bath than almost anything. The warm water gently disperses the oil and surrounds you in a soothing, healing immersion. Be sure to mix the oils into the water before immersing yourself, so the drops of oil are dispersed. As you soak, your pores open to absorb the hydrating fluid; you inhale the fragrant steam and become permeated with your bath oil blend. Although bathing is considered one of the gentlest applications of aromatherapy, total immersion can have undesirable results if the wrong oils are chosen.

Oils that can be irritating or cause skin sensitivity when added to the bath include citrus oils, cinnamon, peppermint, anise, fennel, and basil.

THE PATCH TEST

If you are unsure of how your skin will react to an essential oil, apply one drop of the oil to the inside of your wrist or forearm. Check the spot for any redness or irritation after a few hours. If you have very delicate skin and wish to be extremely careful, you can cover the spot with a Band-Aid and leave it for 24 hours.

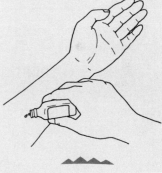

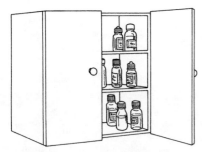

Essential oils should be stored in dark glass containers away from excessive heat and sunlight, and out of the reach of children.

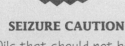

SEIZURE CAUTION

Oils that should not be used by people with epilepsy are:

◆ Fennel
◆ Hyssop
◆ Rosemary

SAFE STORAGE

Oxidation and rancidity of essential oils can also cause toxicity. These may be due to improper storage, exposure to high temperatures, or contamination from other chemicals. Essential oils should always be stored in dark glass containers away from sunlight and heat. The ideal storage temperature is between 60° and 80°F (16° and 27°C). In France 20°C is considered stable.

INTERNAL USE OF ESSENTIAL OILS

Oral use of essential oils has become such a controversial subject lately that I feel strongly about taking a stand on it.

There is more and more information being spread about internal use and my feeling is if people are going to self-administer, it is better to have the advice from a professional therapist as to the correct oils to use and the amounts and duration of treatment. That oral use is practiced and can prove beneficial for some people for specific purposes cannot be ignored.

Most of the English books on aromatherapy don't encourage internal use. Aromatherapy is usually part of a massage or a bath treatment or an inhalation. Until recently the English aromatherapists did not advocate the use of aromatic diffusers or some of the other French methods.

In France internal use of essential oils has been accepted and used for a long time. New discoveries have been found in more effective ways of internal usage. It has been found that using a good excipient like olive oil, for example, is a more efficient system of delivery to the mucous membrane, dispersing the oils over a larger surface area. This is especially effective when dealing with infections and viruses that require stronger measures.

Whether you are administering essential oils safely in low dilutions through the skin, or placing essential oils in suppository form

TREATING EMERGENCIES

Olive oil is the solvent of choice for diluting an oil burn. If an essential oil is accidentally splashed in the eyes or on sensitive skin, immediately douse the affected area with olive oil. This acts as an absorbent fat, binding to the essential oil, diluting its effects, and enabling removal. Other vegetable oils or aloe vera gel can be used as an alternative to olive oil. Never use water to dilute an oil burn; it will only disperse the essential oil, increasing the area of damage.

If a dangerous quantity of essential oil should be accidentally ingested, act immediately by drinking olive oil. Then induce vomiting. The olive oil will dilute the essential oil and slow its absorption. Do not drink water, which will only accelerate absorption of the essential oil.

Olive oil and aloe vera gel are good antidotes for an essential oil burn.

rectally, you want to deliver an appropriate amount to have the desirable result. If you feel you don't have enough knowledge or confidence, don't try internal use. Instead become knowledgeable by gathering information and understanding the hows and whys of ingesting essential oils and then consult a qualified aromatherapist for guidance (see page 131).

EMERGING WORLD STANDARDS

The safe use of aromatic materials as perfume and cosmetic ingredients is subject to a voluntary code of ethics that is widely accepted in the aroma industry, a sort of self-imposed honor system. The International Fragrance Association (IFRA), located in Switzerland, acts as a sort of world clearinghouse for safety and quality data. The number of trade groups and independent associations that support research and standardization of aromatic products is growing in countries that have an economic interest in the aroma industry. For example, in the United States the Research Institute for Fragrance Materials (RIFM) gathers information and conducts independent testing of synthetic fragrance preparations, perfume compounds, and essential oils. Its data is subjected to academic scrutiny by a committee of experts on all aspects of composition, safety, and application of fragrance materials, and then submitted to the IFRA to be shared with other such organizations throughout the world.

For books on essential oil safety, see Recommended Reading.

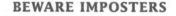

BEWARE IMPOSTERS

It can't be emphasized enough that only genuine essential oils are appropriate for aromatherapy use. There are many wonderfully fragrant synthetic preparations available. Although these synthetics may have many suitable applications, aromatherapy is not one of them. The actions of synthetic preparations are unpredictable and unreliable at best, and can be damaging. Many chemicals found in fragrances are designated hazardous waste chemicals. These include methylene chloride, toluene, methyl ethyl ketone, methyl isobutyl ketone, ethanol, and benzyl chloride. An aromatic product identified on the label as "fragrance" is undoubtedly of synthetic composition.

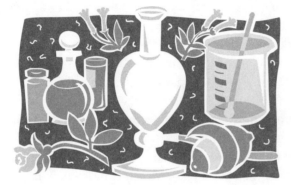

Carrier Oils —
The Vehicles
of Delivery

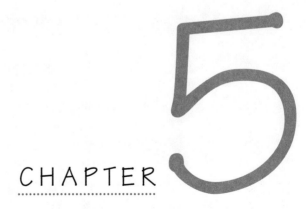

CHAPTER 5

The term *carrier oil* refers to the solution — usually a vegetable oil — in which an essence is diluted. The carrier literally becomes the vehicle in which the essential oil travels, and often serves to slow the action of the volatile oil as well. Carrier oils are fixed oils, meaning they are not volatile. A fixed oil, unlike an essential oil, feels thick and greasy. Carrier oils are sometimes referred to as base oils.

The benefits of essential oils can be undermined if you pay too little attention to selecting your carrier oils. A carrier oil should be carefully chosen for its complementary and synergistic actions. You might choose a carrier oil simply for its feel or scent. You might also consider its nutritional content. Quality should be a major consideration for anything you plan on applying to the skin.

Vegetable oils carry their own vitality and have therapeutic effects of their own. When your main concern is skin care, the choice of carrier oils is of primary importance. For example, if you have very oily skin, you might select hazelnut oil as a carrier for its astringent quality, rather than sesame oil, which is much heavier. Vegetable oils can add nourishment to any type of skin treatment. Rose hip seed, borage, and macadamia nut oils all support the elasticity and suppleness that are important factors in keeping skin healthy and young.

THE MANUFACTURE OF "NATURAL" PRODUCTS

Fats and oils are the primary ingredients used by the cosmetic industry. They serve as emulsifiers, solubilizers, and emollients in creams, makeup, lotions, and soaps. While cosmetic chemists have not historically distinguished between animal and vegetable fats, consumers have begun to reject products manufactured with animal fat as "impure." The response of the cosmetic industry has been to encourage the notion that vegetable-derived products are "pure" products. As a result, a plethora of "natural" beauty products has sprung up around the manufacture of vegetable fat derivatives.

The ubiquitous coconut is one of the major sources of "natural" cosmetics and, perhaps along with other palm kernel derivatives, its use has done more to adulterate the term *natural* than anything else. The slew of synthetic products derived from these fats enables marketing teams to label a product "natural" when it in fact retains little or none of the wholesome quality of the original substance.

Fats and oils are modified, or split into their basic constituents: glycerin and fatty acids. The fatty acids are recovered, distilled, and subjected to further chemical cocktails. The end result is a manufactured item, tasteless, odorless, stable, and neutral. The original botanical name may be retained, but the label really should say "manufactured."

Refinement Is Really Removal

Refining is done for three reasons: to remove the natural fatty acids; to alter or remove color; and to alter or improve taste and odor. The objective of the refinement process is a light, odorless, nonoxidizing, physiologically stable oil with an extended shelf life. In marketing jargon, this process is called "purification." The term *pure* becomes grossly misleading when consumers interpret it to mean that a product has remained close to its natural state.

Oil refining for the food and cosmetic industry follows a few basic steps. It begins when the seed, nut, or other vegetable matter passes through breaking rollers to produce a coarse meal. The meal is cooked until the walls of the oil-retaining cells are burst. Unfortunately, such high temperatures destroy many of the health-promoting enzymes and nutrients. The cooked meal passes through an expeller, which squeezes crude oil, with or without heat, into a tank.

From here it is filtered and bottled. Oils bottled at this stage are generally considered superior and priced accordingly. Marketing literature often refers to the benefits of simple filtration and applied cold pressure, but the original kettling or cooking is obscured.

Further Refinement

Meal left in the expeller still contains oil, which is obtained through solvent extraction. The meal, now pressed into cake form, is dried, flaked or broken, and passed into the extractor. High-pressure jets of solvent wash the oil from the flaked cake in a series of trays at descending levels. As one tray overflows into another, the oil is concentrated. Finally, the mixture is heated and the solvent driven off to be condensed and reused.

In the next step of the refinement process, the oil is heated in a tank, and its natural fatty acids are removed by spraying it with a solution of caustic soda. The acids and alkalis combine to form soap, which sinks to the bottom of the tank and is run off. Further rinsing may take place and the oil may be mixed with fuller's earth, a highly absorbent claylike substance that, when filtered off, leaves a lighter and clearer product. To obtain a neutral quality, hot steam is passed over the oil under a vacuum to lift out any aromatic substances. The end result of this lengthy process is a highly refined oil.

This bland substance is certainly not an ideal choice for use in aromatherapy. It may do the job as a mere carrier for essential oils, but such a manufactured, denatured product contributes very little.

The oil-processing industry exists to meet the demands of major markets: cosmetics, food, soap, and detergents. You can see why virgin, unheated, cold-pressed oil not only is expensive but can be difficult to find as well. As with essential oils, some vegetable oils may carry misleading or confusing labels. If you wish to use a "whole" product, your choices may be very limited.

STORING CARRIER OILS

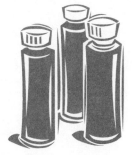

Trust your nose and taste buds to discern the quality of oils. The purpose of refinement is to prolong shelf life and prevent rancidity. Good cooks understand this when they keep their finest olive oil under refrigeration. The same principle applies to your rich carrier oils. When purchasing a good carrier oil, buy no more than you will use in a month or two. Store your carrier oils in a cool cupboard in narrow-necked bottles. Avoid "collecting" carrier oils. Limiting the oils you keep on hand will give you better quality control. Rancid oils should never be used in therapy.

THE VALUE OF UNREFINED OILS

Aromatherapy attributes the benefits of topical application to the permeative power of the oils used. Unrefined oils have an abundance of nutrients that are readily absorbed through the skin.

Essential fatty acids (EFAs) are critically important as the building blocks for cell membranes and intracellular structure. EFAs are also one of nature's most effective moisturizers. Evening primrose, borage, black currant, and flaxseed oils all contain an essential fatty acid helpful in the production of hormones.

Oils rich in vitamins A and E are particularly good for skin conditions such as rashes, allergies, acne, and dermatitis. Although vitamin A is only available from animal sources, carotenoids, substances that are metabolized as vitamin A, are abundantly available from vegetable oils. Much of the color associated with nut and seed oils (yellow/brown) is provided by the carotenoids. The bright orange color seen in CO_2-processed rose hip and carrot seed oils indicates a wealth of beta-carotene (sometimes called pre–vitamin A).

Vitamin E, valued for its antioxidant properties, is found in grapeseed, peanut, sesame, sunflower, and wheat germ oils. It can also act as a preservative when added to other oils. Vitamin C, although water soluble, is another powerful antioxidant found in rose hip seed oil.

The green color characteristic of good olive oil indicates chlorophyll content. Soy oil from unripe beans and rapeseed oil are also rich in chlorophyll. Chlorophyll carries trace amounts of magnesium, which is helpful in treating migraines as well as muscle and joint pain.

Is the Evidence In?

Most of the research done on vegetable oils has examined their nutritional benefits. The effects of topical applications are therefore conjectural. The cosmetic industry recognizes the value of EFAs and is actively funding research to support such conjecture. However, we can only expect cosmetic research to support subcutaneous activity. Proof of systemic activity would necessarily move products from the realm of cosmetics into the medical arena. Therefore, any forthcoming research will most likely remain discreet in interpretation. As holistic practitioners, aromatherapists rely on empirical evidence; we see the benefits in practice. These benefits can only be fully achieved using first-quality oils.

CARRIER OILS USED IN AROMATHERAPY

There are countless wonderful vegetable oils to choose from when you select a carrier oil. Costs vary widely and are primarily a result of where the oil is grown and produced. Purchasing an oil grown or produced regionally is often your most cost-effective choice.

In the United States, for example, almond, jojoba, apricot, peanut, avocado, and safflower are some of the most widely available oils. Canada produces and exports great quantities of canola (rapeseed) oil, and Mexico does the same with coconut. In Europe, grapeseed, hazelnut, and sunflower oils are commonly produced. In the Mediterranean area, olive oil is produced in great abundance. Most sesame oil comes from Asia.

All carrier oils should be kept cool, and even refrigerated in warm and tropical climates. In winter, or in cooler climates, they can be kept in a cool, dark cupboard. Most of the oils in the following list have a maximum shelf life of six months to a year (unless otherwise indicated). Oils kept beyond their shelf life may turn rancid from oxidation or bacterial contamination. Rancid oils have a telltale bitter

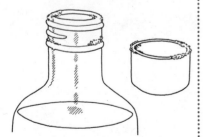

Crystallization around the cap or lip of a bottle of carrier oil indicates the oil has turned rancid.

odor, and bacterial contamination imparts a sour smell. Spoilage is also indicated by crystallizing or solidifying around the lip of the bottle or inside the cap. Spoiled oils should be discarded.

In reality you will have to search hard to find fresh, rich, natural carrier oils. Most oils pass through some sort of cooking process on their way to market. If you want the best quality, buy only "virgin cold-pressed oil." You may even find organic vegetable oils in your health food stores or supermarket.

Remember to buy and store wisely.

ALMOND OIL, SWEET (*Prunus dulcis*)

Sweet almond oil is a light, nongreasy, pale yellow oil obtained through cold pressing almond kernels. It is a wonderful choice as a massage or body oil, my first choice for many years. Midwives traditionally use sweet almond oil for massage of the perineum during pregnancy and labor to prevent tearing. Sweet almond oil is produced primarily in California, Spain, and Italy.

ALOE VERA GEL (*Aloe barbadensis*)

Aloe vera gel is a clear, odorless, nearly tasteless, watery gel with an abundance of healing properties of its own. It is soothing and healing for burns, skin irritations, and raw open wounds.

The gel is easily extracted from the succulent leaves of the plant. A type of lily, the plant has a unique ability to retain water. When the plant is damaged, it seals off the wound immediately, and heals itself quickly. It is an excellent carrier for both oral and topical applications of essential oils.

APRICOT KERNEL OIL (*Prunus armeniaca*)

Apricot kernel oil has a pale orange tint and properties similar to those of sweet almond. The oil is very light, perfect for facial use. It is also an excellent choice as a body or massage oil for skin types that do not accept oils very easily. As the name implies, the oil comes from the kernel of apricot and is widely produced in the United States.

CAUTION

Bitter almond oil should never be confused with, or substituted for, sweet almond oil in aromatherapy. Bitter almond oil and its synthetic twin, nitrobenzene, is the scent of Jergens Lotion, marzipan, and amaretto liqueur. Although it smells wonderful, bitter almond contains prussic acid and can burn sensitive skin.

AVOCADO OIL *(Persea americana)*

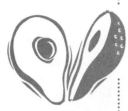

The best-quality unrefined avocado oil is thick, with a rich olive green color. Refined, its color becomes pale yellow. The oil is pressed from the dried flesh and inner peel of the avocado fruit. Avocado oil is rich in saturated and monounsaturated fats, vitamins A, B, and D, and lecithin. It is beneficial to dry, weathered, or wrinkled skin, but due to its thick, heavy quality, avocado oil should constitute no more than 25 percent of a base oil formula.

Avocado has an excellent shelf life because of built-in antioxidants. Much like olive oil, it will thicken if refrigerated. The thickened oil can be liquefied by placing the bottle under hot running water for a few moments.

BORAGE SEED OIL *(Borago officinalis)*

Borage seed oil is clear and thick with very little odor. It contains an abundance of gamma linoleic acid (GLA), an essential fatty acid that the body uses to manufacture prostaglandins — hormonelike substances that balance and regulate cellular activity. Borage seed oil is used both internally and externally. It reduces the aging process of the skin and reverses damage from ultraviolet rays. Borage seed oil is often used to treat premenstrual syndrome, endometriosis, and menopausal discomforts. Herbal tradition prescribes the blue star-shaped borage blossom as a heart tonic and mood elevator.

CANOLA OIL *(Brassica napus* var. *oleifera)*

Also known as Canadian rapeseed oil, canola oil is very light in texture and color. While it is not my first choice for therapeutic purposes, canola is an affordable and versatile oil useful for all skin types. Canola oil is produced on a large scale in Canada and marketed heavily in the United States as a healthful cooking oil.

CARROT SEED OIL *(Daucus carota)*

Cold-expressed carrot seed oil is not to be confused with steam-distilled essential oil of carrot seed. The expressed oil is viscous, pale yellow, and aromatic. Rich in beta-carotene, vitamins B, C, D, and E, and essential fatty acids, carrot seed oil is an anti-inflammatory useful for treating skin rashes, dry skin, and burns. Some people believe that applying carrot seed oil around the eye area will improve eyesight!

CASTOR OIL *(Ricinus communis)*

This thick, heavy, yellowish oil, derived from the castor bean, has a long history of use in folk medicine. Taken internally, castor oil is a strong laxative. Castor oil packs applied with warmed flannel are believed effective for pain relief and to "draw out" cysts, tumors, and warts.

COCOA BUTTER *(Theobroma cacao)*

A hard saturated fat, cocoa butter has a strong, sweet, chocolate scent. An excellent skin softener, it is the perfect oil for massaging daily into fast-growing pregnant bellies to prevent stretch marks from developing.

COCONUT OIL *(Cocos nucifera)*

Coconut oil in its refined state is a stable, inexpensive, and widely used saturated (solid at room temperature) vegetable fat. Coconut oil is also one of the major sources of synthetic detergents. Coconut and its many chemically altered cousins are the bases for countless commercially marketed moisturizers; refined coconut products, however, can actually be drying to the skin. In Mexico, unrefined coconut oil is marketed as *Aceite de coco.* In its raw state, coconut oil is a wonderful product, rich and emollient with a strong coconut scent.

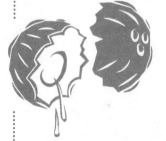

EVENING PRIMROSE OIL *(Oenothera biennis)*

Made from the flowers of the evening primrose, whose blossoms open and glow luminously at night, evening primrose oil is a pale yellow oil with a pleasant, light, and nutty taste. It is rich in gamma linoleic acid (GLA), an essential fatty acid that is vital to cell and body functions and not produced by the body itself. Clinical studies and grassroots research in Great Britain and the United States have demonstrated evening primrose oil's effect as a free radical scavenger and verified its effectiveness in treating endometriosis, menstrual difficulties, high blood cholesterol, and abnormal cell growth in the breasts, ovaries, and uterus. The oil can be used externally, ingested in capsule form, or taken straight (a teaspoon daily).

Some of the many other conditions evening primrose is used for include obesity, arthritis, hyperactivity, alcoholism, premenstrual syndrome, schizophrenia, multiple sclerosis, cardiovascular disorders, hair and skin problems, eczema, and even hangovers. It is also used to induce labor.

FLAXSEED OIL *(Linum usitatissimum)*

Flaxseed oil is made from seeds of the plant that also gives us linen. Flaxseed oil contains essential fatty acids, including omega-3 fatty acids, without which the brain and nervous system cannot function. The metabolic activity of dopamine, seratonin, and insulin are dependent on the presence of omega-3 for optimum function. Flaxseed has a sweet and nutty flavor when fresh, but it deteriorates quickly. The oil can be taken orally (2 tablespoons daily) to support cardiovascular health and as a cancer preventive.

FORAHA OIL *(Calophyllum inophyllum)*

Foraha oil is an opalescent green, slightly waxy oil. It has analgesic, anti-inflammatory, and antibiotic properties. Foraha oil is useful in treating varicose ulcers, adhesions, sciatica, rheumatism, and shingles. The oil, produced in Madagascar is also called "kamani." It comes from a tree of the *Guttiferae* family, which also produces fragrant flowers and fruit. The oil is cold pressed from the seed, which is round and about the size of a macadamia nut.

GLYCERIN *(Olea europaea)*

An odorless, colorless, syrupy derivative of olive oil, glycerin has long been used as a benign solvent, lubricant, and preservative. It is sweet tasting, warming to the skin, and edible. Glycerin is used as an ingredient in edible love oils.

GRAPESEED OIL *(Vitis vinifera)*

The grape seed is tiny and hard with a very low oil yield that is nearly impossible to extract through cold pressure. Even though grapeseed oil is extracted with heat and solvents, next to almond oil it has been my oil of choice for aromatherapy and massage for years. It has a nice "slip" (lubricant quality) and no scent, so it carries delicate floral essential oils without altering their fragrance.

I discovered grapeseed oil in 1995 when a deluge destroyed the California almond crop and doubled the price of sweet almond oil. Grapeseed oil, a by-product of the wine industry, was being marketed at the time as a gourmet cooking and salad oil. I tried it out of desperation and it quickly became my carrier oil of choice. Grapeseed oil is high in vitamin E, which makes it very stable, and it retains traces of picnogenol (OPC), an intense free radical scavenger and antioxidant that has an antiaging affect. In France, the same OPC extracted from pine bark has been marketed for decades as a pharmaceutical product.

HAZELNUT OIL *(Corylus avellana)*

Hazelnuts yield a pale amber oil with a pleasant aroma. Hazelnut oil is important as the only fixed nut oil with an astringent quality, making it beneficial for use on oily skin. It is very popular with German and Swiss therapists.

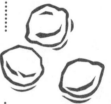

JOJOBA OIL *(Simmondsia chinensis)*

Jojoba is actually a liquid wax extracted from the jojoba bean. Jojoba is very close in nature to human sebum, a natural oil excreted around hair follicles. It can be clogging to the pores for some people. Jojoba oil has replaced the sperm whale oil and "spermaceti" that was used in cosmetics, creams, mascara, and lipstick for more than a century. It has such fine viscosity that it is also used as a machine lubricating oil.

Jojoba oil is incredibly stable, lasting for years without going rancid. Tom Janca has been producing jojoba oil in Arizona since 1973. He sells it unrefined (a golden color) and fine (clear). Janca's slogan is "Grow plants for profit, don't kill for it. Save the whales."

KUKUI NUT OIL (*Aleurites moluccana*)

One of the lightest oils for the face, kukui provides just the right amount of lubrication without leaving a greasy feeling. The kukui nut, native to Hawaii, is high in linoleic acid, and is quickly absorbed into the skin. It is used by the Hawaiians for skin conditioning after sun exposure. It is also a very strong laxative if taken internally, and it has a distinctive odor.

LECITHIN

Lecithin is a mixture of the fatty acids found in all living cells. It protects cells from oxidation and keeps them soft. As an emulsifier, it has the remarkable ability to suspend water in oil. Lecithin is obtained from soybeans or egg yolks. It is used in many cosmetics as a thickener, an emollient, and an antioxidant. It is also thought by some to enhance hair growth.

MACADAMIA NUT OIL (*Macadamia integrifolia*)

Macadamia nut oil, also known as Queensland nut oil, comes from a small evergreen tree native to Australia. Macadamia nut trees are now grown commercially in Hawaii. The oil is high in palmitoleic acid, a monounsaturated fatty acid that acts as an antioxidant, preventing deterioration of cell membranes. For mature skin it is hydrating and gentle. Palmitoleic acid does not occur in any other plant oil, but is found in human sebum. Although macadamia nut oil is expensive, it has a long shelf life.

NEEM OIL (*Azadirachta indica*)

Neem oil is extracted from a plant that grows in India. It is a fixed, waxy, yellow-green oil with a strong toasty aroma. It is used as a moisturizer, as a toothpaste additive, and for nail and cuticle care. In Germany, neem oil is a primary treatment for fungal infections.

OLIVE OIL (*Olea europaea*)

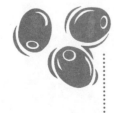

Olive oil ranges from a heavy dark green to a light pale golden color. The intensity of its fruity fragrance and flavor corresponds to its depth of color. The traditional cooking oil of the Mediterranean region, olive oil also has a history as a healing oil. Virgin-pressed olive oil is high in monounsaturated fatty acids, and is helpful in preventing heart disease and high cholesterol. It is also effective for treating constipation, fatigue, hypertension, and rheumatism. Olive oil is the preferred base oil for making salves.

OYSTERNUT OIL *(Telfairia pedata)*

The oil-rich oysternut seed is harvested from the wild in Tanzania. Oysternuts are an important food source for the Tanzanians, who call them *kweme.* The steamed nuts are traditionally fed to a woman immediately after she gives birth, as a tonic, and the oil is massaged into her breasts to increase the flow of milk. Oysternut oil is resistant to rancidity, and rich in iodine and both saturated and polyunsaturated fatty acids.

PEANUT OIL *(Arachis hypogaea)*

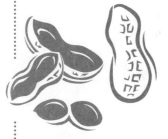

Peanut oil is one of the most widely used oils in the world. It is rich in vitamin E and absorbed easily by the skin. Highly unsaturated, with a strong aroma, peanut oil is nondrying, softening, and conditioning. A hypoallergenic and emollient oil (particularly for arthritis and sunburn), peanut is best mixed 50:50 with a less viscous oil when used for massage. Peanut oil is not very stable in an unrefined state, thus it has a very abbreviated shelf life.

RAPESEED OIL *(Brassica napus)*

Unlike Canadian rapeseed oil (canola), the European variety that is sold as rapeseed oil has a strong, unpleasant smell and is not a good choice for aromatherapy.

ROSE HIP SEED OIL *(Rosa mosqueta)*

Rosa mosqueta grows wild in the southern Andes. Because this environment has not been subjected to chemical fertilizers, pesticides, or fumigants, the natural properties of the flowers are delightfully intact. The bright red hips make a delicious tart jam or rose hip tea. The amber seeds inside the hips contain an oil high in essential fatty acids, GLA, and vitamin C. Dermatologists have found that oil and cream made with rose hip seed oil are excellent for the hair and skin.

In 1978, Dr. Carlos Amin Vasquez reported that he found rosa mosqueta oil superior to any other treatment for seriously burned patients; it caused rapid healing and rejuvenation of skin tissue.

Dr. Fabiola Carvajal has reported superb results using rosa mosqueta oil in clinical studies on scars more than 20 years old, and with patients who had not improved using other therapies. Dr. Carvajal found rosa mosqueta oil beneficial in treating burns, radiation burns, chronic ulcerations of the skin, skin grafts, brown spots, prematurely aging skin, and dry skin.

In Germany, Dr. Hans Harbst has found the same oil to be excellent for postradiation therapy: The application of rosa mosqueta oil produced rapid healing of the inflammation, darkening, and dermatitis caused by radiation. Dr. Harbst also treated cases of severe scarring that had caused tightening of the skin and impaired movement of the extremities. He reported very good results with some patients, and spectacular results with others.

A CO_2-processed rosa mosqueta oil is being produced in Germany. It is very concentrated and retains the tart scent and rich orange-red color of the hips. It is the best antiaging oil I have encountered. According to anecdotal evidence, it is also healing for actinic keratosis and certain early stages of skin cancer.

SAFFLOWER OIL (*Carthamus tinctorius*)

Safflower, along with its relative the sunflower, belongs to the *Compositae* family, the largest family of blooming plants. Safflower seeds have been found in three-thousand-year-old Egyptian tombs. Safflower's orangy yellow flower produces a heavy fixed oil that is high in polyunsaturated fatty acids. Safflower oil can be helpful with a number of circulatory problems when taken internally, and is said to be helpful in treating bronchial asthma. It is also beneficial for painful joints, sprains, and bruises. As a massage oil on its own, I find it rather too thick and sticky. I prefer to blend a small amount with a lighter oil.

SESAME SEED OIL *(Sesamum indicum)*

The seeds of the sesame plant are contained inside a long nut; when cold pressed, they give a high yield of clear, pale yellow oil. Sesame seed oil is rich in vitamins and minerals. Its vitamin E content gives the oil excellent stability. Sesame oil is beneficial for dry skin, psoriasis, and eczema; it also protects the skin, adding warmth and suppleness to the body. Sesame oil is used extensively in Ayurvedic treatments, especially for vata imbalances (see chapter 10).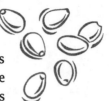

SHEA BUTTER *(Butyrosperum parkii)*

Also called karite butter, shea butter is expressed from the pits of the fruit of the African butter tree. Shea butter is a pinkish, semisolid fat that has gained popularity in massage therapy for foot and body care. It has no smell, and despite its gummy texture it is quickly absorbed to moisturize and nourish the skin.

SOLUBOL

Solubol is a complex vegetable mixture of sunflower oil, water, glycerin, beeswax, propolis, soy lecithin, and vitamin E. It was developed in France specifically as a carrier for essential oils. The creamy lotion is completely oil and water soluble, and the glycerin adds a sweet taste to ease internal use. Solubol is a wonderful addition to the growing array of carrier oils available for aromatherapy.

SOYBEAN OIL *(Glycine max)*

Extracted from the highly nutritious beans, soybean oil is similar in smell to the toasted sesame oil used in Oriental cooking. A rather heavy, strong-smelling oil, it is not one of my personal choices for aromatherapy, but further research may reveal unique properties. Some of the more highly refined soy oils are lighter and not so heavily scented.

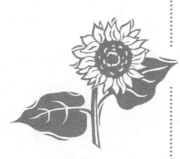

SUNFLOWER OIL *(Helianthus annuus)*

Although most sunflower oil is solvent extracted, some cold-pressed varieties are becoming available. Sunflower oil has a light texture and is pleasant to use, leaving the skin with a satiny-smooth, non-greasy feel. Sunflower oil contains vitamins A, B, D, and E, a high linoleic acid content, and few saturated fatty acids. It is helpful in treating arteriosclerosis, has a protective effect on the skin, and is healing when applied to leg ulcers, bruises, and skin diseases. In Russia, sunflower leaves and flowers are ingested to treat bronchitis and asthma. In France, sunflower oil is one of the primary cooking oils; it is called *tournasol,* which means "turns toward the sun."

WHEAT GERM OIL (*Triticum* spp.)

Wheat germ oil has a rich, orangy brown color. Due to its high vitamin E content, it can be added in small amounts to increase the stability of other oils. Paradoxically, on its own wheat germ oil oxidizes rapidly. It must be kept refrigerated, and still has an extremely short shelf life: 20 to 30 days maximum.

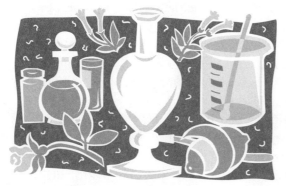

Basic
Aromatherapy
Applications

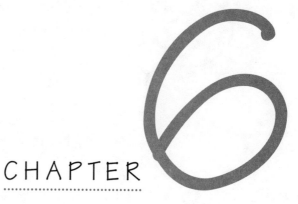

CHAPTER 6

My first profound experience with aromatherapy occurred while treating a severe sunburn — my own. I was in pain and had already tried various sunburn remedies, but nothing helped. When a blend of herbs and oils quickly brought soothing relief, it got my attention. I began to inquire into the properties of various oils and to explore their many possible applications.

Then at the age of 34 I contracted an infectious liver disease. It was a very frightening experience. I was severely ill and my health remained fragile for many months after I had recovered from the most acute stage of the illness. It was during my recovery that I learned to trust in the profound healing power of essential oils. My liver had become so compromised during my illness that my body rejected food and medicines. I'm convinced that the essential oils I used during that time restored my liver to its full function.

There are so many different ways to use aromatherapy in your own life. Essential oils can be applied directly to the skin as part of a massage, reflexology, or meridian treatment. They can be dispersed in a bath, inhaled, or diffused into the atmosphere of a room. They can even be used internally, taken orally under proper supervision, or inserted as a suppository. Specific oils affect specific systems throughout the body. You can target these various systems if you know how to select an essential oil for its properties, and how to select an effective and efficient means of delivery in each case.

BODY AND SKIN CARE

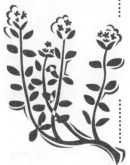

Most of us see our skin as a natural barrier. We imagine that not only does our skin hold us in, but it also keeps everything else out. We imagine that if our skin is unbroken, we present an impermeable surface, immune to the chemical stew of our environment. But our skin, our largest organ, is not impermeable. Acting more like a very fine sieve, our skin "breathes." As it inhales, it absorbs fine traces of the

EFFECTIVE APPLICATION TECHNIQUES
FOR PARTICULAR BODY SYSTEMS

Essential Oil Application	Internal Organs and Systems Affected
Inhalation with diffusers	Respiratory/pulmonary
Internal uses	Digestive/eliminative
Douches and boluses; suppositories	
Bath or spa therapy	Works energetically on organ meridians
Massage and frictions; "aroma glows"	
Algae, seaweed, and thalassotherapy	Endocrine system/skin
Herbal aromatic body wraps; poultices	
Inhalation with diffusers	Neurochemical response
Subtle work: essences, crystals, color lights, homeopathy	Emotional responses

stuff on its surface; as it exhales, chemicals are excreted as fine components of sweat and sloughed-off skin cells.

The outer skin, made up of about 30 layers of cells, is called the epidermis. We shed dead skin cells every day. As the top layer of our skin dies off, a new layer is generated at the base. But as our skin ages, this process of cellular reproduction slows down. If the top layers are not sloughed off, the formation of new skin cells is slowed even further, and the complexion becomes tired and muddy looking.

In 1968, researchers demonstrated the permeability of the human skin by attaching radioactive "tags" to chemicals in cosmetic preparations. The preparations were applied to the skin of human volunteers and the tagged chemicals were later identified in the volunteers' waste products. When I read, nearly 30 years ago, about this study, it changed my attitude about the ingredients I was putting on my skin.

I learned that essential oils placed on the skin are absorbed rapidly. In as little as 5 to 20 minutes an essential oil, applied topically, makes its way into the bloodstream, is carried to the lungs, and is exhaled with the breath. Essential oils are also eliminated through the skin, released in sweat through the pores, and released in urine through the bladder. As the essential oil travels though the body systems, tissues and organs benefit from its healing action.

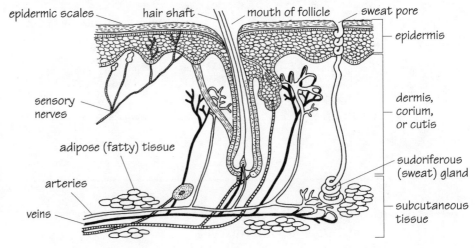

epidermic scales — hair shaft — mouth of follicle — sweat pore

epidermis

sensory nerves

dermis, corium, or cutis

adipose (fatty) tissue

sudoriferous (sweat) gland

arteries

veins

subcutaneous tissue

The skin acts as a sieve, inhaling and exhaling particles. Essential oils applied to the surface eventually make their way into the muscles and bloodstream.

EFFECTIVE ESSENTIAL OILS FOR EACH SKIN LAYER

Skin Layer/Function	Recommended Essential Oils
Epidermis or acid mantle: Strengthen, increase, regenerate, and soften skin	Skin of citrus oils: orange, lemon, grapefruit, mandarin
Dermis or connective tissue: Elasticity, elimination of metabolic wastes, detox, pigmentation	Leaf oils: peppermint, rosemary, thyme, lavender
Subcutaneous or fatty layer	Root oils: vetiver, spikenard

ASTRINGENTS AND TONERS

Astringents and toners are an essential component of any successful facial-cleansing routine. They invigorate the complexion, remove any traces of soap, close up the pores, and quickly restore the skin's protective acid mantle (pH level). Here are several recipes.

HERBAL TONER
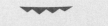

235 ml (1 cup) distilled or spring water
30 ml (1 ounce) witch hazel
2 tablespoons *each* of the following herbs (dried):
    nettles, fennel, coltsfoot, marsh mallow, benzoin gum, comfrey, calendula, peppermint, orange blossoms, eucalyptus, chamomile, lavender, elderberries, lemon peel
12 drops lemon essential oil
12 drops lavender essential oil
30 ml (1 ounce) aloe vera gel
30 ml (1 ounce) glycerin

1. Combine the water and witch hazel in a small saucepan and heat to a simmer.
2. Remove from the heat, add the dried herbs, and allow the mixture to steep for 10 minutes.
3. Add the lemon and lavender essential oils to the herbal mixture and stir.
4. Strain liquid through a cheesecloth to remove herbs. Add the aloe vera and glycerin.
5. Use a small funnel to pour liquid into a dark glass bottle and seal with lid.
To use: Apply to face with a cotton ball or pad to refresh the complexion and remove any residual soap or cleanser.

METRIC CONVERSION MADE EASY

I always use the metric system. Metric measurements are logical units of 10s and 100s that divide easily. You too should become familiar with the metric system, because every country in the world, with the exception of the United States and Britain, uses it.

1,000 ml = 1 liter
480 ml = 16 fluid ounces (1 pint)
60 ml = 2 fluid ounces
30 ml = 1 fluid ounce
15 ml = 1 tablespoon
5 ml = 1 teaspoon
1 ml = 25 drops = 1 gram

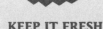
BRISK TONER

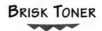

10 drops lemon essential oil
7.5 ml (1½ teaspoons) apple cider vinegar
120 ml (4 ounces) distilled water

Combine all ingredients in a dark glass bottle. Shake well.
To use: Apply to the face and neck after cleansing.

CUCUMBER TONER

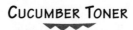

This is a wonderful formula for clarifying the complexion. Use it to feel crisp and clean during hot and muggy weather.

½ cucumber
15 ml (1 tablespoon) lavender hydrosol
30 ml (1 ounce) witch hazel
2 drops rosemary essential oil

1. Combine all ingredients in a blender and blend until the cucumber is liquefied.
2. Strain through a coffee filter or cheesecloth. Put in a dark glass bottle with a lid and store in the refrigerator.
To use: Apply to the face and neck after cleansing.

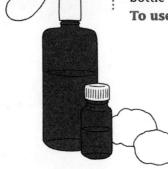

You can make your own toners simply and inexpensively. Store them in dark glass bottles.

BODY TONIC

This is a wonderful tonic for skin that needs firming.

- 2 drops sage essential oil
- 12 drops lavender essential oil
- 10 drops rosemary essential oil
- 5 ml (1 teaspoon) glycerin or solubol
- 120 ml (4 ounces) rose water

1. Dissolve the essential oils in the glycerin or solubol.
2. Combine with the rosewater in a spray bottle, and shake to mix.
To use: Use as a body spray, after bathing, or as an invigorating midday pick-me-up.

AROMA FRICTION

Using blends of essential oils with loofah scrubs or for brushing on dry skin is very energizing and toning.

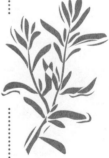

- 5 drops thyme essential oil
- 3 drops savory essential oil
- 12 drops MQV essential oil
- 90 ml (3 ounces) distilled or spring water

Combine the essential oils and water in a spray bottle; shake to mix.
To use: To stimulate and improve circulation, spray onto a loofah or body brush and scrub briskly over your body before or after a morning shower. Stimulate your meridians by working from the foot to the groin area, from the fingertips to the chest, and up the backs of your legs.

FACIAL OILS

Facial oils soothe and nourish the delicate skin of the face. They seal the skin, helping it retain precious moisture and providing protection from surface contaminants. They are also important components of facial massage. By reducing friction, they prevent stretching and wrinkling of the skin.

SENSITIVE OR INFLAMED SKIN LOTION

Formula 1

    2 drops chamomile essential oil
    2 drops neroli essential oil
    7 drops sandalwood essential oil
    5 drops bois de rose essential oil
  30 ml (1 ounce) hazelnut oil

Formula 2

    5 drops geranium essential oil
    2 drops rose essential oil
    5 drops frankincense essential oil
  30 ml (1 ounce) almond oil

Combine all ingredients in a small dark glass bottle and shake to mix.

To use: After cleansing and toning, place a few drops in the palms of your hands and massage lightly over your entire face.

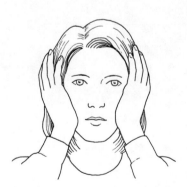

Apply facial oils gently, massaging with the palms of your hands.

Oily Skin Lotion

10 drops niaouli essential oil
5 drops cypress essential oil
30 ml (1 ounce) hazelnut oil

Combine all ingredients in a small dark glass bottle; shake to mix.
To use: After cleansing and toning, place a few drops in the palms
of your hands and massage lightly over your entire face.

Aging Skin Lotion

This wonderful facial formula supports cellular regeneration.

5 ml (1 teaspoon) sage essential oil
5 ml (1 teaspoon) rose geranium essential oil
5 ml (1 teaspoon) lavender essential oil
5 ml (1 teaspoon) rosemary 'borneol' essential oil

Combine all ingredients in a small dark glass bottle; shake to mix.
To use: After cleansing and toning, place a few drops in the palms
of your hands and massage lightly over your entire face.

Moisturizing Lotion

3 drops vetiver essential oil
5 drops orange essential oil
10 drops lavender essential oil
30 ml (1 ounce) almond oil

Combine all ingredients in a small dark glass bottle; shake to mix.
To use: After cleansing and toning, place a few drops in the palms
of your hands and massage lightly over your entire face.

Bust-Firming Lotion

5 ml (1 teaspoon) lavender essential oil
10 ml (2 teaspoons) calendula oil
10 ml (2 teaspoons) St.-John's-wort oil
40 ml (1⅓ ounces) wheat germ oil

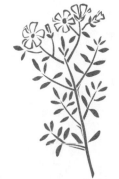

Blend all ingredients; store in a dark glass bottle.
To use: Massage a small amount of oil over the entire bust area after your shower or bath for a youthful and glowing look. Follow up with a spritz of Body Tonic (see page 93).

Choosing Essential Oils for Your Skin Type

Skin Type	Recommended Essential Oils
Acne and congested	Thyme (sweet), neroli, bergamot, tea tree, spike lavender, sandalwood, jasmine, everlasting, mandarin
Normal	Lemon, jasmine, rose, lavender, chamomile
Dehydrated	Carrot, rosemary 'verbenon', neroli, sandalwood, inula, everlasting
Oily	Melissa, lemon, lemongrass, basil, eucalyptus (E. radiata), camphor
Mature or Wrinkled	Myrrh, frankincense, angelica, cistus, spikenard, violet, galbanum
Fragile, sensitive, allergic	Bulgarian rose, blue artemis, blue chamomile, lavender

THIGH FLAB LOTION

40 ml (1⅓ ounces) almond oil
20 ml (4 teaspoons) jojoba oil
10 drops carrot essential oil
12 drops cypress essential oil
10 drops juniper essential oil
20 drops lavender essential oil

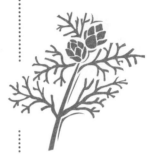

Blend the almond and jojoba oils in a 120 ml (4-ounce) dark glass bottle. Add the essential oils and shake to mix.
To use: Begin with a dry friction massage, scrubbing the flabby area briskly with a loofah or body brush. Follow up by massaging this blend into the warmed and invigorated skin.

POSTWAX BLEND

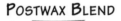

10 drops lavender essential oil
 5 drops marjoram essential oil
 2 drops blue chamomile essential oil
20 ml (4 teaspoons) wheat germ oil
40 ml (1⅓ ounces) apricot oil

Combine all ingredients in a 60 ml (2-ounce) dark glass bottle and shake well to mix.
To use: Apply after waxing to calm and soothe irritated skin and prevent follicle infection.

The Seven-Step Facial

Practiced weekly, this facial care program will cleanse and revitalize a dull complexion.

1. Cleanse. You can use the mild soap or cleanser of your choice.

2. Exfoliate. I keep a jar of homemade cleansing grains in my bathroom — a simple mixture of equal parts oatmeal, cornmeal, and ground almonds. Take about one tablespoon of the grains in the palm of your hand, add a little warm water to form a paste, and gently scrub your face and neck. Allow the grains to set on your face for a few minutes, then rinse with warm water, or rub off gently with your fingertips.

3. Steam. Heat at least 2 liters (2 quarts) of water to a simmer and pour into a large basin or bowl. Add 2 to 4 drops of an essential oil of your choice. Lean your face over the steaming water and drape a bath towel over the back of your head, forming a tent to capture the steam. Be careful not to burn yourself. Relax and let the fragrant steam engulf your head for 5 to 10 minutes.

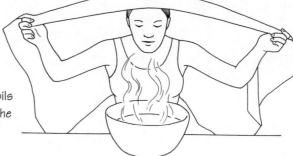

A facial steam with essential oils added to hot water opens up the pores and relaxes the soul.

4. Massage. Gently *pat* your face dry — don't rub it. Choose a facial oil blend and sprinkle a few drops into your palms. Rub your palms together and massage lightly over your face. Starting at the base of your neck, massage up your throat in a sweeping motion to your chin. From the corners of your nose, sweep under your cheekbones and up to your temples. Smoothing across your forehead, continue around your ears to the back of your neck, then down over your neck, shoulders, and bust area.

5. Mask. Choose one of the healing clay masks listed in the box on page 100. Apply to your entire face and neck, avoiding your lips and around your eyes. Apply thickly to any areas congested with pimples or blackheads. Leave on for 20 minutes and then remove with a moistened washcloth.

6. Tone. Apply the toner of your choice (see pages 91–92) to clarify your complexion, close your pores, and remove any residual clay.

7. Moisturize. Top off your facial with a light application of a moisturizer or facial oil blend. In a few hours, your face will be glowing with health and vitality.

CLAY MASKS, PACKS, AND POULTICES

Clay is one of the oldest of all skin treatments. Its cleansing and soothing properties were probably discovered by the women of ancient Egypt as they bathed along the banks of the Nile. Clay contains an abundance of silica and other mineral salts. Silica is a natural mineral that can take many forms, and acts as a carrier of catalysts in chemical reactions. It is present in sand and glass, and is found in the human body wherever hard edges appear, such as in the skin, nails, and hair.

Clay is a balancer and revitalizer. When applied to the skin as a mask, oxidation and circulation are accelerated, defensive functions are stimulated, and body temperature is raised.

Clay has certain little quirks that are important to know about. Dry clay powder can be stored easily. It is often sold in paper packaging, and no harm will come if dry clay is stored in plastic. However, as soon as water is introduced, the clay is activated; from this point it should come into contact only with organic materials.

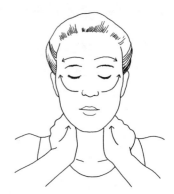

For the most effective massage, follow the paths indicated by arrows with the palms of your hands.

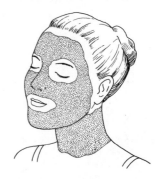

A healing clay mask draws out impurities and nourishes the skin.

HEALING CLAY MASKS

Mix a few drops of essential oil into 1 ounce (30 g) of wet clay to create a healing mask.

Green clay is an excellent all-purpose clay for healing and cleansing. It can be used both internally and externally.

Rose clay is highly absorbent and thus more drying. It makes an excellent cleansing mask.

White clay is very light and pure; used in its dry form, it is an excellent base for body powders.

Yellow clay contains sulfur compounds. It is used to make clay packs to promote the healing of broken bones as well as to treat bone pain, sprains, and muscle aches and strains.

Ideally, this means mixing and storing in glass or ceramic vessels. Wet clay doesn't agree with plastic, and combining clays with metals can set off unpredictable and undesirable chemical changes.

Use wooden spoons or chopsticks for mixing and stirring, and make sure the water you use is pure. You don't want to apply a clay mask to your face with bacteria growing in it! Distilled water is your best assurance of purity, but a reliable hydrosol or spring water can enhance the action of a clay mask. Measure your dry clay into a ceramic bowl and stir in enough water or hydrosol to form a soft paste. Add a few drops of an essential oil of your choice and mix thoroughly.

Use only healing clays found in a health food store. The type of clay used for ceramics is not advised. Leave the clay mask on until dry, then wash off with warm water or scrub off for an exfoliation treatment.

Clay packs and poultices can also be used to treat pains and sprains, to promote the healing of broken bones, and to draw infections or foreign objects to the surface of the skin. When you're using a clay pack to treat pains, sprains, or broken bones, covering it with plastic wrap will retain moisture longer.

Spot Treatment

To treat a solitary, emerging pimple, place a drop of tea tree oil directly on the blemish. Then moisten the tip of your finger with water and dip it into a package of dry rose clay. Dab the moistened clay onto the pimple to make a "mini poultice" and leave overnight.

Drawing Poultice

Measure a small amount of dry yellow clay into a ceramic bowl. Stir in enough water to make a peanut-butter-like consistency. Add a few drops of cypress. Apply the poultice over a stubborn sliver and leave on overnight. Its drawing action will pull the sliver to the surface for easy removal. You can also use this to draw out a small infection.

AROMATHERAPY FOR PROBLEM CONDITIONS

The antibacterial and antifungal properties of essential oils make them ideal for preparing gentle treatments for nagging problems.

FOOT DEODORANT POWDER

    2 drops sage essential oil
    2 drops coriander essential oil
    2 drops spearmint essential oil
225 g (8 ounces) white clay powder
    1 tablespoon baking soda

Combine the essential oils with the clay powder and baking soda in a widemouthed jar. Stir thoroughly.

To use: Powder your feet after bathing and before retiring at night. Sprinkle the powder in your shoes to prevent odor.

CORN AND CALLUS TREATMENT

    4 drops benzoin essential oil
   12 drops lavender essential oil
    6 drops myrrh essential oil
   60 ml (2 ounces) almond oil

Combine all ingredients in a 60 ml (2-ounce) dark glass bottle, cover, and shake to mix.

To use: Massage oil into your feet to soften corns and calluses.

FOOT RELIEF

Another treatment for corns and calluses is to paint the problem spot with the sticky resin of Peru balsam, then cover with gauze. Leave for a day and remove with alcohol. The corn or callus will loosen and be more easily removed.

CANDIDA BLENDS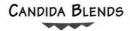

Some women are tormented by chronic vaginal yeast infections. A yeast infection is actually the result of an overgrowth of a beneficial organism: *Candida albicans,* which is present throughout our bodies, only causes problems when it grows unchecked by our system's natural defenses. Aromatherapy offers a pleasant, safe, and effective means of reestablishing a healthy balance as well as relieving the unpleasant symptoms of yeast overgrowth. The following blends are all effective for treating yeast. Let your choice be governed by your scent preference, your intuition, or the availability of ingredients.

Formula 1

2 drops tea tree essential oil
2 drops spike lavender essential oil
2 drops bois de rose essential oil

Formula 2

2 drops palmarosa essential oil
2 drops neroli essential oil

Formula 3

2 drops tea tree essential oil
2 drops oregano essential oil

Formula 4

2 drops lavender essential oil
2 drops tea tree essential oil
2 drops myrrh essential oil

Combine the essential oils in the selected formula in a small dark glass jar.

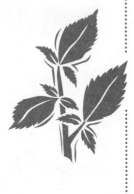

To use candida blends:

- Take the blend orally by mixing 2 to 4 drops in a cup (235 ml) of warm water, or an ounce (30 ml) of solubol. (Caution: see page 131 regarding oral use.)
- Use the blend vaginally with a silk cosmetic sponge soaked in a warm, sterilized-water solution. You can purchase from your druggist a sterile "silk," or natural sponge, that will work quite well. Tie a length of dental floss to the sponge, leaving a 4-inch (10 cm) "tail" for convenient retrieval.

   Disperse the essential oils blend into a cup (235 ml) of warm, sterilized (previously boiled) water. Immerse the sponge. Gently squeeze out the excess moisture — so it is not dripping — and insert the sponge into the vagina, leaving it overnight. You can wear a sanitary pad for security.
- Use the blend vaginally in a bolus. Also called ovules, boluses are female vaginal suppositories that are used to treat vaginal infections. You can easily make your own with a cocoa butter base.

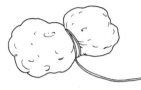

A sterile silk or natural sponge can be used to make a vaginal insert for treating yeast infections.

COCOA BUTTER BASE BOLUS

60 ml (2 ounces) cocoa butter
30 g (1 ounce) white clay
   Essential oil blend of your choice for candida (see page 102)

Melt the cocoa butter over low heat. Add the clay and essential oils. Chill the mixture in the refrigerator until the cocoa butter just begins to harden. Form in boluses, about the size and shape of the tip of your little finger. Place on a sheet of wax paper in the refrigerator. When they have hardened, store in an airtight glass container in the refrigerator.

To use: Insert one bolus vaginally each night before bed. Continue treatment until symptoms disappear.

KELOID AND SKIN TAG TREATMENT

   5 ml (1 teaspoon) everlasting essential oil
   5 ml (1 teaspoon) sage essential oil
15 ml (1 tablespoon) rose hip seed oil

Combine the everlasting and sage with the rose hip seed oil in a 1-ounce (30 ml) dark glass vial and shake to mix.
To use: To reduce or remove keloids and skin tags, apply 1 or 2 drops directly to the area several times a day.

HERPES FORMULA I

   5 drops everlasting essential oil
   5 drops niaouli essential oil
30 ml (1 ounce) St.-John's-wort oil (olive oil maceration)

Combine the everlasting and niaouli essential oils with the St.-John's-wort in a 30 ml (1-ounce) dark glass vial; shake to mix.
To use: Apply this blend to active herpes lesions to speed healing and relieve discomfort.

HERPES FORMULA II

   2 drops rose essential oil
   2 drops melissa essential oil
   5 ml (1 teaspoon) honey
235 ml (1 cup) warm water

Stir all ingredients together. Mix well.
To use: Drink once a day until symptoms clear up. (See caution regarding internal use on page 131.)

Herpes Formula III

10 drops basil essential oil
10 drops geranium essential oil
30 ml (1 ounce) olive oil

Combine all ingredients in a small dark glass bottle and shake to mix well.

To use: Rub into your ankle or sacrum area to arrest the viruses within the nerve root.

Shingles Blend

5 drops Roman chamomile essential oil
2 drops peppermint essential oil
10 drops lavender essential oil (*Lavandula angustifolia* ssp. *angustifolia*)
5 drops eucalyptus essential oil (*Eucalyptus radiata*)
30 ml (1 ounce) St.-John's-wort oil (olive oil maceration)

Combine all ingredients in a 30 ml (1-ounce) dark glass vial and shake to mix.

To use: Apply this blend to painful areas to soothe aggravated nerve endings and speed healing.

Rash Reliever

10 drops German chamomile essential oil
30 ml (1 ounce) aloe vera gel

Combine the ingredients in a widemouthed glass jar and mix well.

To use: Apply to irritated areas.

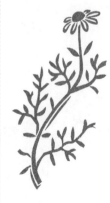

Scleroderma Treatment

2 drops spikenard essential oil
10 drops lavender essential oil
5 drops lemon essential oil
5 drops orange essential oil
30 ml (1 ounce) grapeseed or almond oil

Combine the essential oils with the grapeseed or almond oil in a small dark glass vial and shake to mix.

To use: Apply this blend to soften hardened and thickened areas of the skin, and elsewhere to discourage abnormal fibrous tissue growth.

Eczema Blend

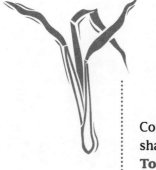

5 ml (1 teaspoon) lavender essential oil
5 ml (1 teaspoon) lemongrass essential oil
10 ml (2 teaspoons) foraha essential oil
30 ml (1 ounce) rose hip seed oil

Combine all ingredients in a 60 ml (2-ounce) dark glass bottle and shake to mix well.

To use: Massage this blend into inflamed areas to soothe and speed healing. In cases of chronic recurring eczema, massage this blend onto sites where the inflammation first occurs to prevent and decrease flareups.

HYDROSOLS

Hydrosols (also called flower waters and hydrolats) are by-products of essential oil production. They are produced during the distillation of essential oils. The waters used in the distillation process become naturally scented and impregnated with the plants' subtle water-soluble properties. Traditionally packaged in blue glass bottles in France, flower waters have been produced and used in cooking and cosmetics since ancient times in the Middle East, Tunisia, Egypt, and India. Jeanne Rose, executive director of the Aromatic Plant Project, has popularized herbal hydrosols in North America. She notes this is a more accurate term than flower waters, since many are made from leaves, bark, or other parts of the plant.

The name *hydrosol* comes from the Latin *hydro* (water) and *sol* (sun). One pound of plant material can yield 1 quart of aroma-impregnated water. Of every 5 gallons of water used in distillation, maybe 1 to 1½ gallons are recovered as a hydrosol product.

The process of steam distillation using aromatic plants creates two complementary products: the essential oil and the hydrosol. Following the cooling of the aromatic gas, the oil-soluble components separate from the water. As they separate they pass on part of their qualities and a small percentage of themselves: Maybe 2 to 10 percent of the essential oil ends up in the hydrosol.

Hydrosols present themselves as perfect companions to such alternative health therapies as phytotherapy and homeopathy, and are excellent for people who are too sensitive to use essential oils.

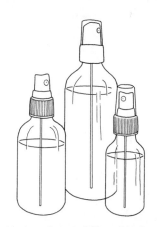

Hydrosols are diffused with this type of pump bottle, often available in dark blue glass to protect the oils from sunlight.

HYDROSOLS RECOMMENDED FOR SKIN TYPES AND SPECIAL USES

Skin Type/Use	Hydrosols
Normal skin	Neroli, rose, lavender, rosemary
Dry skin	Rosemary, orange blossom, rose
Oily skin	Melissa, lemon verbena, inula
Mature skin	Rose geranium, everlasting, rose
Eye compresses	Myrtle, elder flower, chamomile

Herbal hydrosols make excellent toners and skin refreshers. Those currently produced and commonly available in the United States and France include:

Bulgarian rose

Eucalyptus

Everlasting

Hyssop

Inula

Lavandin

Lavender

Lemon verbena

Linden

Melissa

Moroc rose

Myrtle

Neroli

Orange blossom

Peppermint

Rose geranium

Rosemary

Rosemary 'verbenon'

Turkish rose

Thyme

My Personal Favorites

I first learned to appreciate the effects of hydrosols while traveling at night from San Francisco. During the two-hour drive I would stay alert by spritzing myself. Hydrosols kept me alive many times. I never travel without a bottle of rose water. My interest in hydrosols has led to some interesting experiments with homemade hydrosol stills. In my first attempts, I put a recycled water purifying distiller to work. My distillation adventures with friends around different places in California have resulted in some very special hydrosols.

Artemisia douglasiana

This special water is steam distilled in Oregon and California from the plants *Artemisia douglasiana* and *A. californica.* These plants — also called wild mountain sage — are similar to Indian sage, commonly used for "smudging," a sacred ritual used by the Native North Americans to clear negative energy and purify the air. The Indians used cedar, sage, and artemisia along with many other scented herbs. An elder Native woman once explained to me that the sacred smoke carried their prayers to the Great Spirit.

I have found this floral water to be very beneficial for either skin that is too dry or skin rashes that will not heal. It is refreshing and invigorating when sprayed on the face and body.

Lippia citriodora (lemon verbena)

The leaves for this herbal hydrosol, also know as *Aloysia triphylla,* were hand-harvested from a 25-year-old tree in Jeanne Rose's Victorian garden in San Francisco and brought to Mendocino, California, to be distilled in July 1992, by Hubert Germain Robin. Hubert is a third-generation French master cognac distiller. I arrived in Mendocino after a three-hour drive and emerged into the green hillsides of Hubert's property. When I entered his immaculate still house, I was enthralled by an old copper piece of equipment used by alchemists.

I noticed Hubert's pale lavender T-shirt and was reminded of the French alchemist Saint Germain, who was called "The Master of the Violet Ray." Naturally scented with the plants' subtle water-soluble properties, this hydrosol is lovely for the skin, and very calming to the psyche.

Achillea millefolium (yarrow)

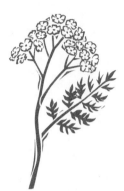

Yarrow blossoms were first wildcrafted from the beautiful and wild Big Sur coast of California in the summer of 1994. The distiller, Karl Lee, is also an alchemist, trained by Albertus. The power and strength of this water is remarkable. Yarrow flowers have many uses in traditional herbology.

Native North Americans drank a tea made from yarrow. They used it for purifying the skin before sweats and saunas, for it has the ability to raise the body temperature. In spiritual and psychic work, yarrow is used as an aura shield and protector from negative outside influences. Yarrow contains tiny water-soluble chemicals that do not reduce into the essential oil; it also contains sesquiterpenes, which make the hydrosol very soothing to the skin. In Russia yarrow was experimented with to combat the aftereffects of radiation from the Chernobyl incident.

The hydrosol can be used in its natural state as a spray, or it can be diluted in distilled water and used as a detoxifying drink; 10 or 12 drops is sufficient.

Pelargonium graveolens (rose geranium)

Some hydrosols are now being been commercially produced in California as part of a grassroots wildcraft aromatherapy movement that started in the 1980s. The plants that produce the rose geranium hydrosol, for instance, are grown in Sonoma, California, for the Aromatic Plant Project. The project was organized by Jeanne Rose, who originally set out to get farmers, grape growers, and gardeners to grow lavender in various parts of California, especially those areas from 2 to 20 miles inland of the Pacific Ocean.

HYDROSOL BLENDS

I created the following hydrosol blends while working in a skin clinic. They are the result of my own observation and study of the French concepts of skin care and hydrosol blending.

VELLEDA

30 ml (1 ounce) Roman chamomile hydrosol
30 ml (1 ounce) rose geranium hydrosol
60 ml (2 ounces) Bulgarian rose hydrosol

Mix the waters together in a 120 ml (4 ounce) plastic spray bottle and shake.
To use: Misting the face with this blend works to rejuvenate on a deep cellular level. The effect is more profound with mature or aging skin. It is also good for very sensitive skin and imparts a natural glow.

HYDRA

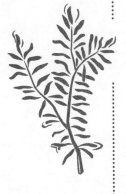

30 ml (1 ounce) rosemary hydrosol
60 ml (2 ounces) French lavender hydrosol
30 ml (1 ounce) neroli hydrosol

Mix the waters together in a 120 ml (4 ounce) plastic spray bottle and shake to make a rare and beautiful water solution.
To use: This blend is lovely for the skin and calming to the psyche; it maintains skin freshness if yours dries easily or if you live in a dry climate.

Naiad

60 ml (2 ounces) lavender hydrosol
30 ml (1 ounce) sweet thyme hydrosol
15 ml (1 tablespoon) melissa hydrosol
15 ml (1 tablespoon) lemon verbena hydrosol

Mix the waters together in a 120 ml (4 ounce) plastic spray bottle and shake.

To use: Naiad is useful for overactive sebaceous glands, blemishes, acne, and problem skin types.

Delphi

30 ml (1 ounce) Bulgarian rose hydrosol
30 ml (1 ounce) rose geranium hydrosol
60 ml (2 ounces) lavender hydrosol

Mix the waters together in a spray bottle and shake.

To use: This blend is energizing, for a fast pickup when you need mental and physical energy to perform your best. It also rejuvenates the skin.

More Hydrosol Combinations

The following blends can be prepared in whatever quantity you need. Just mix together in a plastic spray bottle and shake.

Dry Skin Blend
1 part rosemary 'verbenon' hydrosol
1 part thyme 'linalol' hydrosol

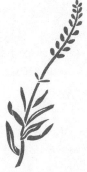

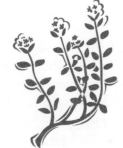

HYDROSOL APPLICATIONS

All hydrosols can be applied with a cotton ball or pad directly to the skin, or by misting 10 to 12 inches from the face with an atomizer. These spray bottles come in different sprays, from a fine mist to a squirt; choose one with a fine mist.

Hydrosols are perfect for use while traveling, especially during air travel, which is dehydrating. Hydrosols are also refreshing in the car, and in drier climates, which dehydrate the skin. Occasional sprays have kept me awake during late, long-distances drives.

Hydrosols can also be used in making perfume, eau de Cologne, or toilet water.

Acne Blend
- 1 part thyme hydrosol
- 1 part lavender hydrosol
- 1 part neroli hydrosol

Sensitive Skin Blend
- 1 part lavender hydrosol
- 1 part chamomile hydrosol
- 1 part *Artemisia arborescens* hydrosol

Rejuvenating Blend
- 1 part rose geranium hydrosol
- 1 part rosemary hydrosol

Soothing Blend
- 1 part lavender hydrosol
- 1 part rose hydrosol
- 1 part thyme hydrosol

Oily Skin Blend
- 1 part lavender hydrosol
- 1 part lemon verbena hydrosol
- 1 part *Artemisia* hydrosol

BALNEOTHERAPY

Balneotherapy is the art of water therapy, and one of aromatherapy's best friends. There is nothing quite so soothing and relaxing as a leisurely soak in a hot bath. As the warmth of the water cradles your physical body, providing relief from the constant pull of gravity, your psyche is refreshed and restored, the weight of the world momentarily lifted. Add a few drops of well-selected essential oils and you approach nirvana.

Water is nature's greatest and most effective solvent. It acts as a liquid suspension, carrying a variety of minerals and chemicals, depending on its source. When we immerse our bodies in a warm bath, our skin rapidly begins to absorb chemicals that are suspended in the water. These chemical components can make their way to our bloodstream in as little as 2 to 15 minutes. It will take a normally healthy person from half an hour to three hours to eliminate most of these chemicals through the expired breath and urine. In unhealthy or obese people, this process may take up to 10 hours. That is why adding essential oils to a bath is such an effective aromatherapy treatment.

The premise of balneotherapy is built on this solvency. Just as we absorb the essential oils we intentionally add to the water, we absorb a variety of other chemicals and minerals suspended in our water. No two waters are exactly the same. Spring waters, often thought of as pure, actually contain a variety of minerals. It is the presence of these minerals, from the depths of the earth, that makes certain spring waters highly valued for their curative properties.

The amazing virtues of water have been sung throughout the ages. Ancient myths featured countless sea nymphs, mermaids, and water goddesses. It's no wonder that most ancient gods and goddesses associated with water were believed to be sources of life, fertility, and fecundity. Water is our element. We most likely evolved from aquatic creatures — and in any event, our first months of life were spent floating in an amniotic bath. In our dreams water symbolizes the ebb and flow of our emotions. We use water for cleansing, refreshing, and relaxing. Water is the basis for our body's evaporative cooling system. It flushes out toxic wastes, plumps up our cells, and lubricates our moving parts. Water is crucial to our survival. Without it we would literally dry up and blow away.

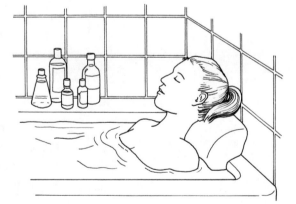

The bath is one of the simplest and most enjoyable ways to enjoy aromatherapy.

A Brief History of the Bath

Although the Romans may not have invented the bath, they raised bathing to a high art. Roman citizens lingered for hours in communal hot baths, where they socialized, conducted courtship, and even sealed business deals. They built lavish baths wherever they found natural hot springs. The remains of Roman baths are still evident throughout Europe, the Mideast, and North Africa.

The Roman reverence for bathing has survived in Turkey, where patrons still visit public baths to be soaped, steamed, and scrubbed clean by attendants. Meanwhile, a highly ritualized bathing culture has evolved in Japan as well. Whole towns exist as destination resorts around Japanese natural hot springs. The harried Japanese make annual visits to these springs, and in between find time for frequent visits to the "Sento" — the local communal hot-tub house. Japanese homes are for the most part poorly heated, and the family bath becomes an important source of warmth in winter.

With the fall of the Roman Empire, bathing fell out of favor in Europe. For the next few centuries the practice was considered suspect and unhealthy, immersion a frightening and distasteful experience. Washing was an unpleasant and infrequent necessity, to be carried out quickly and furtively, with a basin of cold water.

Water Therapy

Water therapy as practiced today was introduced in Austria in the 19th century by the Reverend Father Sebastian Kneipp. Father Kneipp believed in the healing properties of water and prescribed treatments that included drinking mineral waters, soaking in hot springs, taking cold showers, and walking barefoot in the early-morning dew. Healing spas that subscribed to Father Kneipp's philosophy sprang up all over Europe, and "taking the waters" became a popular social pastime for the rich and privileged.

Today health spas abound throughout the United States, Europe, and the Mediterranean. Modern spas have evolved beyond mere mineral-water treatments to offer many other complementary therapies as well as physical fitness, relaxation training, and nutritional counseling. Aromatherapy has been universally adopted as a valuable synergistic component of most spa therapies.

You can create your own spa experience with just a few oils and a tub of hot water. An aromatherapy bath is the ultimate luxury. Experiment with 3 to 5 drops of several different, complementary oils, adjusting the total amount to suit your individual taste. You can add

COMPLEMENTARY ESSENTIAL OILS FOR THE BATH

Following are combinations of essential oils that you might try for the bath.

Soothe Your Worries Away
Lavender
Chamomile
Geranium

Floral Escape
Rose
Bois de rose
Ylang ylang

Pampered & Scented
Bois de rose
Frankincense
Clary sage
Geranium

Luxurious Soak
Roman chamomile
Angelica
Neroli
Clary sage

Deep Forest Pool
Pine
Rosemary
Eucalyptus

Escape to the Woods
Sandalwood
Neroli
Cedar

Vitality
Ravensara
Thyme
MQV

Very Calm Night Soak
Marjoram
Cypress
Lavender

Longevity Bath
Rosemary
Spike lavender
Oregano

the oils directly to the bath or, for added luxury, disperse them in a cup of milk first. Essential oils combine well with all other bath additives. Add Epsom salts, sea salts, and algae to mineralize the water and increase buoyancy. Add oatmeal or honey to soothe and nourish the skin. Add bicarbonate of soda to "soften" the water. Add fresh or dried herbs and flower petals for their aesthetic and therapeutic qualities.

Thalassotherapy

Thalassotherapy is water therapy with the addition of elements from the sea, mainly seawater and algae. The theories of thalassotherapy are based on the premise that there exists a physiological similarity between the ocean and blood plasma. Our blood does contain certain minerals, notably potassium, sodium, and chlorine, in the same proportions as seawater. It is believed that by warming seawater to body temperature, negative ions are activated; these penetrate the body, bringing the vital elements of the sea to our every organ.

The remineralizing benefits of thalassotherapy are considered to be especially effective in restoring elasticity to sagging skin due to aging or sudden weight loss, or following a pregnancy.

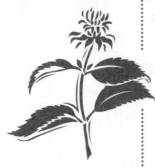

Thalasso treatments can be undertaken at home by soaking in a bath to which has been added 2 to 4 ounces (60 to 120 ml) of algae powder. Besides restoring healthy skin texture, algae soaks promote healthy blood circulation, reduce cellulite and water retention, and soothe sore muscles.

Essential oils that work synergistically with algae powders include cypress, artemisia, lavender, lemon, petitgrain, bergamot, thyme, and juniper.

Algae Bath

This aromatherapy algae bath is particularly beneficial to people who are undergoing strong drug therapies.

120 ml (4 ounces) algae liquid
60 ml (2 ounces) algae powder
4 drops thyme essential oil
5 drops juniper essential oil
2 drops artemisia essential oil
10 drops lavender essential oil

Combine all ingredients in a blender and liquefy, adding water as necessary.

To use: Stir the algae mixture into a hot bath and soak for at least 20 minutes. A weeklong regime of this detoxifying bath daily is very helpful following chemotherapy treatments or surgery, or after any severe illness treated with a strong drug therapy.

A FEW WORDS ON WATER

Drinking and bathing in high-quality water is the most natural way to hydrate your body and preserve and promote your good health. Most tap water from public water supplies is loaded with chlorine, and often laced with other chemicals as well. Some of these chemicals are intentionally added to protect our health — fluoride, for example, is a highly controversial additive intended to harden children's teeth and prevent tooth decay — but other chemicals slip through in minute particles as traces of environmental pollution. If your skin is dry or irritated after bathing, and particularly if you notice a white residue on your skin, you might want to invest in a water filtration system.

MASSAGE

A well-selected essential oil formula enhances any type of massage or bodywork. There are many great books on massage, and hands-on courses are available in most major cities. I believe massage is best learned and practiced with another person. You can glean a lot of practical information from reading about it, but you need to feel and touch to really develop massage techniques. If you are inexperienced and feel insecure about giving or receiving a massage, I have included some tips to help you. Whatever the level of your massage training, aromatherapy can be added. By including essential oils you will enhance the pleasure and therapeutic benefits of the treatment.

When using essential oils in a massage treatment, always choose oils that the person receiving the massage finds agreeable to smell. If you are going to experiment with your own blends, keep in mind that a 2 to 4 percent solution (7 to 20 drops of essential oil to each ounce, or 30 ml, of carrier oil) usually makes an appropriate concentration for a massage oil. Limit your blends to no more than three or four different essential oils. One ounce (30 ml) of massage oil is more than enough for an average massage, unless you are massaging a very large, dry, muscular, or hairy person.

Some Basic Massage Tips

◆ Make sure the room is a comfortable temperature. A warm, well-ventilated room is preferable. Music and soft lights or candlelight can enhance the atmosphere.
◆ Find a still point within yourself before you begin. Start by centering yourself, breathe evenly and deliberately, and feel the weight of your body through the soles of your feet. Feel your energy as it rises through your body, from your feet to your fingertips.
◆ Greet your massage recipient with a soft voice and gently make contact.

SORE MUSCLES OR FATIGUE

Rosemary makes a great massage oil for sore muscles or fatigue, and it blends well with lavender and geranium. Rosemary oil must be diluted before applying to the skin. Add 20 drops to 1 ounce (30 ml) of carrier, or add 15 to 20 drops to bathwater.

- Start slowly, using gentle, long, smooth, connecting strokes.
- Pay attention to muscle knots, constricted breathing, and soft sighs. Take note of painful spots as well as pleasure sites.
- Refrain from chatter. Follow your recipient's lead in conversation and don't be offended if she doesn't talk at all.

HORMONAL CHANGE AND REGENERATION FORMULA

15 drops *Pinus siberian* essential oil
15 drops *Pinus pinaster* essential oil
 3 drops summer savory essential oil
 2 drops angelica essential oil
60 ml (2 ounces) solubol or carrier oil

Combine all ingredients in a small dark bottle and shake well.
To use: Add to a bath or apply as a massage oil.

SENSUALITY BLEND

2 drops jasmine essential oil
2 drops rose essential oil
2 drops sandalwood essential oil
2 drops ylang ylang essential oil
2 drops clary sage essential oil
30 ml (1 ounce) hazelnut oil

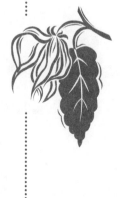

Combine all ingredients in a dark glass bottle and shake well.
To use: Add to a bath or apply as a massage oil.

ESSENTIAL OILS FOR EMOTIONAL AND PSYCHOLOGICAL WELL-BEING

There are numerous ways to choose essential oils for massage. Because massage is such an effective way of transcending emotional barriers, I like to choose massage oils for their psychological effects.

Emotional Challenge	Essential Oils to Aid the Process
Anger (to soothe)	Chamomile, ylang ylang
Anger (unexpressed)	Rosemary
Anxiety	Bergamot, citrus oils, melissa
Apathy	Patchouli
Depression	Clary sage, bergamot, jasmine
Suicidal	Clary sage
Insomnia	Marjoram, neroli
Lethargy	Spruce, pine
Digestive trouble	Fennel, peppermint, cinnamon
Fear	Geranium, juniper, hyssop
Grief	Amber, ylang ylang, rose, marjoram
Grief (in children)	Mandarin orange, peppermint
Low self-esteem	Rose
Loss/death	Cypress, ud, spikenard
Mental stress	Basil, citrus oils, neroli
Calming	Sandalwood, lemongrass, lavender
Physical pain	Ylang ylang, clary sage, birch, spikenard
Oversensitivity	Mimosa, bois de rose
Spiritual/psychic protection	Frankincense, yarrow
Stress	Lavender, geranium, bergamot

Aroma Points and Meridians

Electromagnetic nerve channels run all through the body. The energy of life, known in the orient as *chi* or *qi,* runs along these channels, or meridians. Although chi is difficult to explain, it is real and can be felt. I have felt chi come through my hands while practicing Tai Chi. I have felt it shoot up my spine in deep yoga practice. The concept of this unseen and immeasurable energy, while new to the West, has ruled Eastern thought for centuries. Acupuncture treatments work on a knowledge of chi and its pathways, or meridians.

The Chinese say that chi comes into the body with the breath, then flows through the 12 paired channels called meridians. The meridians can become blocked. Excessive heat or cold can deplete or cause excess energy. Through pulse diagnosis, these patterns can be understood. Symptoms are seen as specific expressions of an organ meridians' state of balance or imbalance. The acupuncturist's task, whether he uses needles or acupressure, is to rebalance the chi.

Volatile in nature and electromagnetic in composition, essential oils have important, subtle psychological and physiological properties. If you accept the concept of chi and acknowledge the healing power of essential oils, it becomes clear that essential oils influence the chi. Through study, conjecture, intuition, and practice, I have identified some specific oils for their balancing effect on the organ meridians.

I have also explored chi pulse correlations to specific patterns in music. For example, I have found that musical chords in the key of A major and B major exert an influence on the gallbladder and liver meridians. The growing awareness and acceptance of vibrational medicine opens an exciting realm of possibility in the relationships of scent, sound, and color and their relationships to the meridians.

Essential oils are very powerful chemical messengers that definitely affect the meridians. Even if you don't understand the concept of meridians or acupressure, you can benefit by rubbing your hands and feet with selected oils.

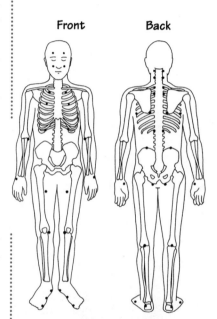

Front   **Back**

These diagrams show the location of meridian (or Jin Shin) points (indicated by black dots) used in traditional Japanese medicine practices of acupressure and acupuncture to stimulate and balance the energy flow in corresponding areas of the body. Applying massage oils to these points can be beneficial as well.

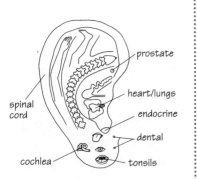

Meridians on the ear correspond to various organs and body parts.

There are numerous acupressure meridians on the face. The gall-bladder meridian starts at the outside corner of the eye, winds around the ear, and down the side of the head, tracing a shape like a Greek war helmet. Sinus and allergy problems originate here, and balancing this meridian can clear the sinuses and the eyes. The stomach meridian runs through the center of the cheek and nose area, and all the way down to the feet. Dry lips and a stuffy, sometimes bloody nose are indications that the stomach meridian is out of balance. Some TMJ problems can be helped by balancing this meridian. The bladder meridian starts at the forehead, near the hairline over each eye, and runs straight back over the crown of the head to the nape of the neck. It continues down the back, where it splits into two forks that run all the way down each side of the spine. The small intestine meridian also runs through the face, along the smile line, from the corner of the nose down to the chin. Breakouts and rashes along this line can indicate food allergies and digestive or eliminative problems.

Other meridians, such as the heart/kidney and spleen/liver, show up on the hands and feet instead of the face. However, all organs are represented on the tongue, in the iris of the eye, and in the ear points.

According to reflexology theory, points on the hands and feet stimulate corresponding body parts, as noted in these diagrams.

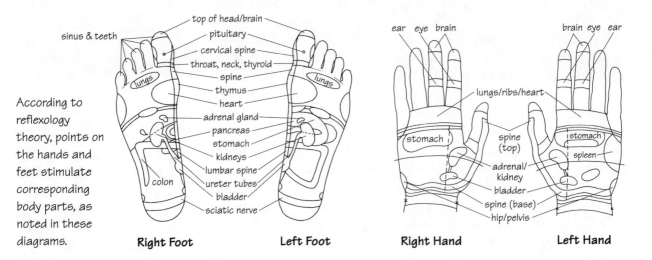

RECOMMENDED ESSENTIAL OILS FOR ADDRESSING MAJOR ORGAN MERIDIANS AND CORRESPONDING EMOTIONS

Organ Meridian	Essential Oils*	Emotions/Attitudes
Lung/Large Intestine	Peppermint Pine Eucalyptus Inula	Grief and sadness. Possessiveness is the principal cause of grief and results in all kinds of accumulations such as cysts and tumors.
Heart/Small Intestine	Melissa Ylang ylang Anise Lemon verbena Rose	Trying too hard, pretending you're okay when you're really not. You don't grow old from laughing! Joy is the positive side of all emotions.
Stomach/Spleen	Fennel Dill Roman chamomile Kewda	Worry is payment on a debt never owed. Obsession, thinking too much, overanalyzing.
Gallbladder/Liver	Rosemary Neroli Rosemary 'verbenon' Lemon Peppermint	Anger, resentment, bitter frustration. Encourages compassion and understanding. A deep laugh helps release anger and fears.
Kidney/Bladder	Juniper Geranium Sandalwood Cedarwood	Fear. Where fear exists, love is absent. Where love exists, there is no fear.
Umbilicus/Diaphragm	Inula Lavender Ud Frankincense Spikenard	A combination of all emotions. Fear of death.

*Use singly diluted or in combinations of 2–3 oils.

AIRBORNE SCENT

One of the miracles of aromatherapy is its absolute simplicity. Just a whiff of the right oil can adjust your attitude, clarify your thinking, steady your resolve, even ease your pain. I'm rarely without a small vial containing some blend to help me through the day. Lavender is often in my pocket for brief inhalations whenever stress is beating me down. A whiff of lemon invariably clears my head and refreshes my thought processes. Inhalations are a practical way to incorporate aromatherapy into your day.

JET LAG INHALATION
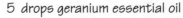

    5 drops geranium essential oil
    5 drops bay laurel essential oil
    5 drops lavender essential oil

Combine the oils in a small glass vial with a tight stopper.
To use: Carry a vial in your pocket or purse while traveling. Sniff periodically throughout your day to forestall the exhaustion and brain fog of jet lag.

STRESS BUSTER #1

Stress wreaks havoc on the immune system. This blend helps boost the immune system.

    5 drops niaouli essential oil
    5 drops ravensara essential oil
  10 drops lavender essential oil

Combine the oils in a small glass vial with a tight stopper.
To use: Carry a vial in your pocket or purse and sniff periodically.

Stress Buster #2

This is a very calming blend.

  5 drops lavender essential oil
  2 drops Roman chamomile essential oil
  4 drops ylang ylang essential oil

Combine the oils in a small glass vial with a tight stopper.
To use: Carry a vial in your pocket or purse to sniff periodically throughout your day.

Media Overload

  5 drops clove essential oil
  3 drops nutmeg essential oil
 10 drops sandalwood essential oil

Combine the oils in a small glass vial with a tight stopper.
To use: Carry a vial in your pocket or purse. As you're working at a computer terminal for extended periods, sniff periodically throughout your day.

The Aromatic Diffuser

There are many ways of scenting an environment. Incense has been used to deliver scent for thousands of years. More recently candle burners, simmering potpourri pots, and lightbulb rings have all become popular methods of dispersing scent atmospherically. Although these methods are aesthetically pleasing, they are not the best choices for aromatherapy. Commercial incense and potpourris are often rounded out with synthetic scents; their purity is unreliable. Additionally, incense smoke may transmit harsh, and even carcinogenic, chemicals along with its pleasing aroma. Candle burners and lightbulb rings can overheat delicate essential oils, changing their chemical makeup.

Diffusers act quite differently. Without altering or heating oils, they disperse them into the environment via an air jet pump connected to a glass bell. A nebulizer within the glass bell diffuses a fine mist of negatively charged, scented ions into the atmosphere, much the same way that nature spreads fragrance.

The aromatic diffuser first appeared in Paris in 1960, when Dr. Bidault demonstrated the germicidal action of aromatic essences on tuberculosis, whooping cough, and influenza. His clinical observations indicated that disinfection of the air surrounding a patient had a therapeutic preventive effect. At the University of Paris School of Pharmacy, students tested his theories by collecting samples of air from an urban factory, the forest of Fontainebleau on the outskirts of the city, and from a Parisian flat. By diffusing various essential oils into sealed chambers containing the air samples, they were able to validate the effectiveness of the essential oils against airborne bacteria and molds.

The modern aromatic diffuser is a natural alternative to aerosol deodorizers and chemical air fresheners. A diffuser is a safe and convenient method of dispersing essential oils throughout a home, school, or workplace.

By using a diffuser, it is possible to dispense a therapeutic aromatherapy treatment to a number of people simultaneously. It is an exellent way of purifying the environment as well as administering the uplifting, rejuventating, or relaxing effects of selected oils or blends to a group.

In the home environment, the therapeutic effects of diffused oils on the respiratory system are especially helpful during the cold and flu season, because the diffuser destroys airborne bacteria. When outside air is polluted, a diffuser can help create a safe, peaceful, and uplifting atmosphere indoors.

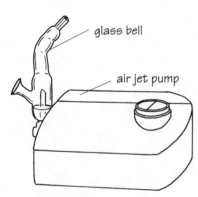

glass bell

air jet pump

A diffuser such as this one pumps a fine mist of essential oils into the air without heating them (which can destroy their effectiveness).

HEALTHY BREATH BLEND

20 drops eucalyptus essential oil (*Eucalyptus radiata*)
20 drops lavender essential oil

Combine the oils in the diffuser receptacle.
To use: Run diffuser for two to four hours in the evening, or all night on a low setting.

GRIPPING COUGH BLEND

20 drops eucalyptus essential oil (*Eucalyptus radiata*)
20 drops ravensara essential oil (*Ravensara aromatica*)

Combine the oils in the diffuser receptacle.
To use: Run diffuser for two to four hours in the evening, or all night on a low setting.

DIFFUSER BLENDS FOR SPECIAL PURPOSES

For	Blends
Respiration	Eucalyptus, lavender, inula
Clean air	Lavandin, lemon, MQV
Purifier	*Thymus 'linalol'*, *T. vulgaris*, lemon
Cold and flu blend	Oregano, lavender, eucalyptus, thyme, clove, cinnamon, peppermint
Calming	Lavender, marjoram, geranium, chamomile
Nervous tension	Lemon, orange, neroli
Meditation	Clary sage, fir, cedar
Depression	Bergamot, geranium, clary sage
Aphrodisiac	Ylang ylang, patchouli, neroli

Bronchial Asthma Blend

5 ml (1 teaspoon) hyssop essential oil
5 ml (1 teaspoon) rosemary 'verbenon' essential oil
5 ml (1 teaspoon) ammi essential oil
2 ml (½ teaspoon) blue chamomile essential oil

Combine the oils in a small dark glass vial with a tight stopper and shake to mix.

To use: Use this blend in a diffuser during flareups of asthma. The blend can also be carried in a small glass vial in the pocket to be sniffed frequently throughout the day.

Asthma with Nervousness and Allergies Blend

5 ml (1 teaspoon) mandarin essential oil
5 ml (1 teaspoon) tarragon essential oil
5 ml (1 teaspoon) rosemary 'verbenon' essential oil

Combine the oils in a small dark glass vial with a tight stopper and shake to mix.

To use: Use this blend in a diffuser during flareups of asthma. The blend can also be carried in a small glass vial in the pocket to be sniffed frequently throughout the day.

Bronchitis with Mucus Blend

5 ml (1 teaspoon) eucalyptus essential oil
5 ml (1 teaspoon) Eucalyptus dives essential oil
5 ml (1 teaspoon) MQV essential oil

Combine the oils in a small dark glass vial and shake to mix.
To use: Use this blend in a diffuser to inhale until mucus is cleared.

Detoxification Blend

10 ml (2 teaspoons) lemon essential oil
5 ml (1 teaspoon) rose geranium essential oil
5 ml (1 teaspoon) everlasting essential oil

Combine the oils in a small dark glass vial and shake to mix.
To use: Use this blend in a diffuser when detoxifying or working on breaking a smoking, alcohol, or drug habit. This blend can also be carried in a small glass vial in the pocket to be sniffed frequently throughout the day.

Heart and Lung Blend

5 ml (1 teaspoon) lavender essential oil
3 ml (¾ teaspoon) angelica essential oil
2 ml (½ teaspoon) *Inula graveolens* essential oil

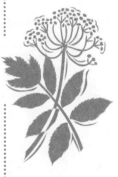

Combine the oils in a small dark glass vial and shake to mix.
To use: Use this blend in a diffuser for two to five hours, preferably at night. Or use an automatic timer to turn on the diffuser at 4 A.M., when the lung meridian is at its high cycle.

Cold and Flu Prevention Blend

5 ml (1 teaspoon) lavender essential oil
5 ml (1 teaspoon) eucalyptus essential oil (*Eucalyptus globulus*)
3 ml (¾ teaspoon) ravensara essential oil (*Ravensara aromatica*)
2 ml (½ teaspoon) bay laurel essential oil

Combine the oils in a small dark glass vial and shake to mix.
To use: Use this blend in a diffuser during cold and flu season.

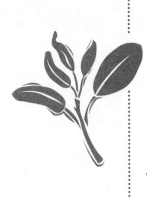

RELAXATION BLEND

 5 drops mandarin petitgrain essential oil
10 drops mandarin essential oil
20 drops lavender essential oil (*Lavandula angustifolia*)

Combine the oils in a small dark vial and shake to mix.
To use: Use in a diffuser to encourage relaxation.

MEDITATION BLEND #1

 4 drops myrrh essential oil
 5 drops sandalwood essential oil
10 drops frankincense essential oil
 2 drops clove essential oil
 2 drops cistus essential oil
 5 drops clary sage essential oil
 2 drops rose essential oil

Combine the oils in a small dark glass bottle and shake well.
To use: Add to a diffuser and use to support and enhance meditation.

MEDITATION BLEND #2

10 drops clary sage essential oil
 4 drops vetiver essential oil
 2 drops cistus essential oil
20 drops cedarwood essential oil
 5 drops fir essential oil

Combine the oils in a dark glass vial and shake well.
To use: Diffuse to support and enhance meditation.

ORAL USE OF ESSENTIAL OILS

The oral use of essential oils has been a subject of great controversy. Most aromatherapists, particularly in the United States, have dealt with the issue by avoiding it altogether.

The political power of, and dominance over the health care industry by, the American Medical Association and the pharmaceutical industry causes aromatherapists to tread very softly in this area. Although you are free, if you choose, to use essential oils internally, an aromatherapist practicing in the United States is unlikely to direct you to ingest any essential oil. That would come dangerously close to practicing medicine. (See also Safety and Toxicity, pages 68–69.)

In France and Germany, the therapeutic use of essential oils has been the subject of much research and attention by the medical community. It is not unusual in these countries for a physician to prescribe oral doses of pharmaceutically pure essential oils to treat many conditions that are routinely treated with antibiotics elsewhere in the world. In contrast, throughout the United Kingdom aromatherapy has been primarily viewed as a cosmetic and aesthetic therapy, and oral use has not been widespread.

Many essential oils, however, are safe to ingest in limited amounts (2 to 3 drops in a carrier or excipient). The commercial food industry uses them abundantly as flavoring agents, and the FDA provides a food-grade rating to indicate purity and safety. These commercially available aromatic oils are all rated "food grade." Many are not even pure essential oils, but rather compounds made up of synthetic fragrances mixed with oils of questionable quality. These oils have no therapeutic effect, should not be used for aromatherapy applications, and should certainly never be ingested!

As our world becomes smaller, and information circles the globe in seconds, books are printed in translation, and aromatherapists get training overseas, a discussion of oral use is becoming unavoidable. As people learn about essential oils and wish to take advantage

CAUTION ON INTERNAL USE

If you wish to use essential oils internally, I advise you to educate youself thoroughly, not only on the general subject of aromatherapy but also on the specific oil you intend to use. Proper dosing is crucial. Just as a single aspirin can work wonders, an overdose can kill. Many essential oils pack a lot more power in a single drop than several ounces of the same herb. The issue of cumulative doses must also be thoroughly understood. (See page 65.)

of their potential healing power, the issue inevitably evolves from a question of therapists insulating themselves from potential legal problems to one of educating the public to prevent them from self-administering potentially toxic doses.

Dispersed in an Excipient

The most current research shows that assimilation of orally ingested essential oils occurs primarily in the duodenum and the first third of the intestinal tract. No digestion of fats occurs in the stomach. Absorption of the active ingredients in essential oils occurs on contact with the surface of mucous membranes. The surface of contact of 1 drop of essential oil is very small, whereas dissolving the oil in an excipient, such as vegetable oil, solubol, glycerin, or honey, and then dispersing it in water greatly increases the surface of contact. Therefore, for efficacy as well as safety, oral doses should always be taken in an excipient.

External Use Results in Internal Effect

That said, I would like to emphasize that any application of essential oils ultimately results in an internal effect. Whether the oils are inhaled, absorbed through the skin, ingested, or supposited, their effect is no less internal. Transdermal application is generally safe and extremely effective. More and more conventional medicines are being delivered transdermally, because it is now understood that by circumventing the digestive system and the liver, smaller doses become effective and cumulative toxicity is less of a danger.

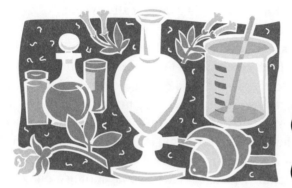

Creating Your
Own Blends

CHAPTER 7

For many people, this is the most creative and fun part of aromatherapy. Here is where you coordinate your senses to create a bit of magic. I love to paint, and I find that the pleasure of creating unique essential oil blends is similar to the pleasure of painting. The whole experience of blending essential oils echoes the tactile delight of choosing my pigments, thinning them with linseed oil or turpentine — the carrier — and blending colors to create a unique palette that I can use to express my creative vision.

When I first began to make my own blends, I had some early successes, and I definitely made my share of expensive messes. Over the years both results have taught me a lot about working with oils. I've learned that in order to create a cohesive blend I must start with a need, a specific purpose. I ask myself, "What am I making the blend for?" "Who am I making it for?" and "What does she need?"

When I teach, beginning students are usually very eager to experiment with the many different essential oils. Although it might be fun to arbitrarily pick and choose oils, adding a pungent scent here to a yummy scent there, the results of such casual blending are often an expensive disappointment. I urge students to ask themselves, "What do I wish to accomplish with this blend?" If they begin with a clear idea, with a need to fulfill, they can be guided by the properties of the essential oils, and begin their blending in the true spirit of aromatherapy. I recommend starting off with simple blends, using no more than three oils in each formula.

GETTING STARTED

When you are creating an original blend, three crucial factors to consider are proportion, property, and intensity.

Proportion refers to the relative quantity of each ingredient. To achieve correct proportioning, you will need to know how to figure a percentage formula.

Property refers to the action of each of the oils in your blend. You should choose oils for their complementary action as well as their scent.

Intensity refers to the relative strength of an essential oil's scent. Some oils can be overpowering when used in very small quantities. Refer to the Odor Intensity Guide on page 145.

Materials

Most of these pieces of equipment can be found at a store that sells essential oils, or a medical supply shop.

Bottles. You will need bottles of different sizes, including several glass bottles that will hold 4 ounces (120 ml). If you are uncomfortable using glass in the bathroom — around a tile tub or shower, for instance — plastic will do for short-term storage of your blends. Plastic, however, will absorb the essential oils over time. You can observe this process when the plastic begins to droop after several months.

Mixing Bowls. You can use glass or ceramic mixing bowls. Glass laboratory beakers are ideal for mixing.

Measuring Devices. Use glass laboratory pipettes or eyedroppers for metering drops. A glass measuring cup marked with ounces will work fine for measuring larger quantities.

Stirring Sticks. I usually use wooden chopsticks. Glass rods work well also.

Essential Oils. You should have several all-purpose oils to begin your blending exercises.

Carrier Oils. Almond is an excellent choice as an all-purpose carrier oil.

You'll need a variety of bottles, bowls, and measuring devices to blend essential oils.

The Percentage Formula

The percentage formula will help you determine the appropriate relative quantities of the ingredients in your blend. It requires a little bit of math, so it might be helpful to keep a calculator handy.

Using the metric (milliliter) system, 1 milliliter equals 20 drops, and 30 milliliters equal 1 ounce. To determine how many drops of essential oil you will need to add to your carrier to create a specific percent solution, you need to first determine the amount of the carrier oil.

For example, using the equivalents I just listed, you can determine that your 1 ounce of carrier is equivalent to 600 drops. If you wish to create a 2 percent solution, multiply 600 by 2 percent (0.02), and you will find that a total of 12 drops of essential oil added to 1 ounce of carrier will create a 2 percent solution. Quantities for a 5 percent solution can be determined by multiplying the 600 drops by 5 percent (0.05), arriving at 30 drops of essential oil to 1 ounce of carrier. It's really that simple!

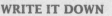

DROPPER EQUIVALENCY FORMULAS

20 drops = 1 ml   30 ml = 1 oz.

To determine the number of drops in your carrier, use this formula:
Total ml carrier x 20 drops per ml = carrier drops
   For example: 1 oz. = 30 ml x 20 drops = 600 drops
                4 oz. = 120 ml x 20 drops = 2,400 drops

To determine number of essential oil (EO) drops, use this formula:
Total carrier drops x percent = drops to add
   For example: To make a 2% solution using 1 oz. of carrier, multiply 600 drops x 2% = 12 drops of EO
   To make a 4% solution using 4 oz. of carrier multiply 2,400 drops x 4% = 96 drops of EO

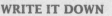

WRITE IT DOWN

Count drops carefully, and consistently record how many drops of each essential oil you use. Experiment with proportions. Keep a card file on your blends. It is a tragedy to make a wonderful blend and lose it because you didn't write it down.

Exercise #1: Blend a Basic Massage Oil

In this exercise you will make a basic massage oil. The ingredients are all gentle oils that blend well, so you really can't go wrong. This blend will make a very gentle and comforting oil. A massage with this oil, for instance, might be soothing for a sick child.

As you introduce your essential oils to the carrier, be sure to mix well, by either shaking or stirring, after the addition of each oil. Count your drops carefully, adding a total of 20 to 30 drops of the four essential oils to your carrier. Adjust the proportions to suit your own taste. Note that the chamomile is very intense and must be used in a lesser proportion than the other oils or it will overpower your blend.

Exercise #2: Blend a Detoxifying Massage Oil

In this exercise you will make a diuretic, detoxifying massage oil to use on cellulite or during weight loss. It would also be appropriate for massage to relieve the discomfort of fluid retention that often accompanies premenstrual syndrome, colds, flu, or overindulgence in food or drink.

As you introduce your essential oils to the carrier, be sure to mix well, by either shaking or stirring, after the addition of each oil. Count your drops carefully, adding a total of 20 to 30 drops of the three essential oils to your carrier. Adjust the proportions to suit your taste.

Exercise #3: Blend an Analgesic Massage Oil

In this exercise you will make a soothing, analgesic massage oil. It would be appropriate for massage to relieve muscle aches and pains that might follow a particularly intense workout. This is a much stronger oil and would not be appropriate to use on young children.

RECORD OF YOUR PERSONAL BLEND #1

Oil	Amount
Carrier — almond oil 4 oz. (120 ml)	
Lavender	_____ drops
Geranium	_____ drops
Clary sage	_____ drops
Chamomile	_____ drops

RECORD OF YOUR PERSONAL BLEND #2

Oil	Amount
Carrier — grapeseed oil 4 oz. (120 ml)	
Cypress	_____ drops
Juniper	_____ drops
Lemon	_____ drops

RECORD OF YOUR PERSONAL BLEND #3

Oil	Amount
Carrier — _____	
	1 oz. (30 ml)
Rosemary	____ drops
Pine	____ drops
Birch	____ drops
Chamomile	____ drops

RECORD OF YOUR PERSONAL BLEND #4

Oil	Amount
Carrier — _____	
	1 oz. (30 ml)
_____	____ drops
_____	____ drops
_____	____ drops
_____	____ drops

You will start with just 1 ounce (30 ml) of a carrier oil of your choice, and add a total of 24 drops of essential oil to make a 4 percent solution. Remember to mix well, either shaking or stirring, after the addition of each oil. Count your drops carefully, and adjust the proportions to suit your taste. Note that the chamomile is very intense and must be used in a lesser proportion than the other oils or it will overpower your blend.

Caution: If you, or anyone who will use this oil, are subject to seizures or have high blood pressure, substitute lavender for rosemary in this blend.

Exercise #4: Create a Relaxing Blend

In this exercise you will blend four oils of your own choice, selected for their scent and action, to make a relaxing and nurturing massage oil. Start with 1 ounce (30 ml) of carrier — almond or grapeseed oil — and add a total of 24 drops of essential oil to make a 4 percent solution.

If you would like a stronger blend, you can add more essential oil. If you would like it milder, you can dilute it by carefully adding more carrier. The strength of the blend and proportions of the essential oils are purely matters of personal preference.

Caution: Always be aware of the possible and probable actions of any oils you add to your blend.

SYNERGY IN BLENDS

When something has achieved synergy, it has become greater than the sum of its parts. Synergy is the reason we create blends. As specific, complementary essential oils merge in a blend, their actions are enhanced; the oils, working in unison, create a more powerful effect.

Exercise #5: Create a Stimulating Blend

White flower oil, a popular Chinese liniment, is traditionally made with eucalyptus, camphor, peppermint, cinnamon, clove, and lavender. Select four of these oils and experiment with relative proportions to create your own stimulating massage oil blend. This will be a strong oil, warming and analgesic, to relieve tired, sore muscles and promote healthy circulation.

Start with 1 ounce (30 ml) of carrier — almond or grapeseed oil — and add a total of 30 drops of essential oil to make a 5 percent solution.

If you would like a stronger blend, you can add more essential oil. If you would like it milder, you can dilute it by carefully adding more carrier. The strength of the blend and proportions of the essential oils are purely matters of personal preference.

Caution: This massage oil will not be suitable for use on children. Always be aware of the possible and probable actions of any oils you add to your blend.

Exercise #6: Create a Pregnancy Blend

In this exercise you will make a mild massage oil (less than 1 percent solution) to be used during pregnancy. Select three oils from those listed in chapter 13 as safe for use during gestation. You might choose to blend a soothing and comforting massage oil, a spiritually uplifting body oil for use with creative visualization, or an oil to moisturize the skin and allay the development of stretch marks. By limiting your choice to the supersafe, user-friendly oils listed as safe for pregnancy, you really can't go wrong.

Start with 4 ounces (120 ml) of almond oil for your carrier. Be sure to shake or stir as you introduce each essential oil to the carrier. Count drops carefully, adding a total of 20 to 30 drops of the three essential oils. Adjust the proportions to suit your own taste.

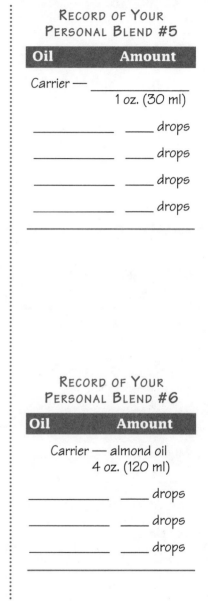

RECORD OF YOUR
PERSONAL BLEND #5

Oil	Amount
Carrier — _____	
	1 oz. (30 ml)
_____	____ drops
_____	____ drops
_____	____ drops
_____	____ drops

RECORD OF YOUR
PERSONAL BLEND #6

Oil	Amount
Carrier — almond oil	
4 oz. (120 ml)	
_____	____ drops
_____	____ drops
_____	____ drops

Record of Your Personal Blend #7

Oil	Amount
Carrier — grapeseed oil 1 oz. (30 ml)	
_____	____ drops
_____	____ drops

Record of Your Personal Blend #8

Oil	Amount
Carrier — _____ 1 oz. (30 ml)	

Bass Note

_____	____ drops
_____	____ drops

Middle Note

_____	____ drops
_____	____ drops

Top Note

_____	____ drops
_____	____ drops

Exercise #7: Create a Children's Blend

In this exercise you will make a simple massage blend suitable for a child. Choose two of the following oils for your blend: lavender, geranium, sandalwood, chamomile, mandarin, neroli, rose, ylang ylang, honey, mimosa. These are all gentle oils that blend well and will combine to make a very soothing massage oil.

Start with 1 ounce (30 ml) of grapeseed oil as a carrier. As you introduce each essential oil, stir or shake to mix well. You will add a total of 12 drops of essential oil to make a 2 percent solution. Count your drops carefully. Note that if you use chamomile, its intensity is overpowering unless it is used in a much smaller relative proportion.

Exercise #8: Blend an Ensemble

In this exercise you will embark on a more complex blending adventure. Taking into account the top, middle, and bass notes, you will create a basic body/massage oil blend using two of the essential oils from each group. Start with 4 ounces (120 ml) of your favorite carrier oil and add a total of 60 drops of the essential oils you chose for top, middle, and bass notes (for a 3 percent solution). Begin by adding your bass notes, mixing after the introduction of each individual oil. Follow with middles and then top notes.

Bass. Select two of the following essential oils to create your bass note: myrrh, patchouli, labdanum, benzoin, Peru balsam.

Middle. Select two of the following essential oils to create your middle note: lemon, orange, lime, bergamot, petitgrain, grapefruit.

Top. Select two of the following essential oils to create your top note: ylang ylang, lavender, bois de rose, rose geranium, palmarosa, chamomile.

Exercise #9: Blend a Perfumed Oil

In this blending exercise you will make a perfumed body oil. Start with 4 ounces (120 ml) of your favorite carrier oil and add a total of 60 drops of essential oils chosen from the top, middle, and bass notes listed below. Begin by adding your bass notes, mixing after the introduction of each individual oil. Follow with middles and then top notes. This exercise will broaden your ability to create balanced formulas with a wider range of oils.

Bass. Choose one of these essential oils to create your bass note: sandalwood, vanilla, amber, patchouli.

Middle. Use all five of these essential oils to create your middle note: bergamot, lemon, orange, lavender, rosemary.

Top. Select one of the following essential oils to create your top note: neroli, rose, jasmine, ylang ylang, cassia.

WORKING WITH RESINS

Resins can be a challenge to work with. Due to their extreme viscosity and tendency to solidify (even distilled resins seek to return to their solid state), resins are difficult to measure. Jojoba oil is a good diluent to thin down resins for use in body and massage oils and oil-based perfumes. Resins also dissolve easily in alcohol.

Warm your resins to thin their consistency and make them easier to work with. Heat about 1 cup (235 ml) of water in a small saucepan. Set your bottle of resin in the warm water, with the cap removed or loosened. In a few minutes the resin will be warmed and of a thinner consistency. Mix 1 part resin to 4 parts of carrier for a sufficient dilute. After gently heating the carrier, the resin can be mixed in by shaking or stirring.

Oil	Amount
Carrier — _____	
	4 oz. (120 ml)

Bass Note

_____ ____ drops

Middle Note

Bergamot	____ drops
Lemon	____ drops
Orange	____ drops
Lavender	____ drops
Rosemary	____ drops

Top Note

_____ ____ drops

Variations on a Theme

Using the basic format you followed in the blending exercises, you can extend your exploration into more complex formulas. The blend you formulated in Exercise #9 can also be blended with a fine-grade alcohol instead of the carrier oil to make a classic eau de Cologne.

A Mary Magdalene Blend

Make an original blend in tribute to Mary Magdalene, patron saint of perfumery, and the archetypal anointer. Begin with 1 ounce (30 ml) of foraha as a carrier oil. Use a bass blend of sandalwood, spikenard, ud, frankincense, and myrrh. Add five middle notes and three top notes of your own choice. Blend in a total of 20 drops of essential oils to make a rich, heady, heavily scented anointing oil.

MAKE A ROSE CREAM

Making this fluffy facial cream can best be compared with making homemade mayonnaise. Measurements, temperature, and timing are crucial. It either works or it doesn't and there's no room for repair when it doesn't work. But don't be intimidated. It's a fairly simple process, and just like mayonnaise, after a few batches you'll be a pro.

This luxurious face cream should last six months. Refrigerate in warm climates.

Materials
3 enamel pots
Wooden chopstick
Medium-size ceramic or glass bowl
Wire whisk
Rubber spatula
60 ml (2 ounce) plastic or glass jar

Ingredients

30 ml (1 ounce) almond or apricot oil
2 g (¹⁄₁₀ ounce) beeswax (do not use paraffin)
30 ml (1 ounce) rose water or distilled water
3 ml (³⁄₄ teaspoon) lemon juice
2–4 drops rose essential oil

1. Warm the almond or apricot oil in one of the enamel pots, and warm the beeswax in another. When the beeswax is melted, stir it into the warm oil with a wooden chopstick.

2. Warm the water in the third pot to the same temperature as the oil-and-beeswax mixture. (It is crucial that the oil and water be very near the same temperature when you mix them. Otherwise the hot oil will spit when it hits the water. The ideal temperature for mixing is 150°F, or 66°C.)

3. Place the warmed water in the mixing bowl and begin whipping with the wire whisk. Drizzle the oil mixture slowly into the water, whipping constantly. Your mixture should cream up quickly.

4. Keep whipping and when the emulsion begins to feel thick, add the lemon juice and the rose oil. Continue whipping until your cream has cooled.

5. With the spatula, scrape the cream into the jar.

Tip: If your mixture stubbornly refuses to emulsify, your water is probably too cold, or your oil mixture too hot. Whipping this cream by hand works better than using an electric beater. If you don't succeed on your first try, don't be afraid to try again. Like making piecrust, it takes a bit of experience to get a feel for your ingredients, and once you've succeeded you'll be thrilled with the results.

You can experiment with the same formula using different floral waters and essential oils. For example, carrot seed oil makes a wonderful cream for aging complexions.

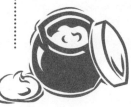

UNDERSTANDING ODOR INTENSITY

The idea of rating odors by their intensity was developed by a cosmetic chemist named Poucher, who worked in London in the 1950s. He was considered by his contemporaries to be the ultimate authority on cosmetic formulation. He proposed rating odors on a scale of 1 to 10 — 1 being the mildest, most fleeting scent, and 10 being the strongest, most permeating scent. This odor intensity guide functions as a tool to help develop well-balanced blends. By considering the intensity ratings of different oils, you can see that you will need more drops of some oils and fewer drops of others to achieve balance. A well-balanced aromatherapy blend, like a music ensemble, should have no single element overpowering the whole. For example: A blend of 10 drops of lavender, 10 drops of bergamot, and 1 drop of blue chamomile will not be well balanced. The chamomile, even in such a small amount, will be overpowering.

Remember, the best guide to blending is your own nose. Develop your sensitivity by working with good-quality oils. Avoid synthetics; they will decrease your nose's sensitivity, as will cigarette smoke.

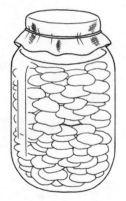

Infused oils are made by using a carrier oil such as almond oil to draw out the essence from the plant material itself.

MAKING AN INFUSED OIL

If you are a gardener or have access to freshly harvested herbs and flowers, you really should try cold-extracting some of your own oil blends. Cold extraction is one of the simplest ways of extracting aromatic oils from plants. It consists of soaking aromatic plants in vegetable oil until their scent has infused the oil. The infused oil can be strained and more plants added, repeating the process until the oil has become sufficiently scented.

I first learned the process from California hippie herbalists in the 1970s. We called it "sun infusion." We collected empty gallon-size pickle and mayonnaise jars, carefully boiled the jars to sterilize

Odor Intensity Guide

Essential Oil	Intensity Rating	Essential Oil	Intensity Rating
Angelica	6	Lemon	3
Basil	7	Marjoram	5
Benzoin	4	Melissa	7
Bergamot	4	Myrrh	6
Black pepper	7	Neroli	5
Blue chamomile	9	Orange	5
Roman chamomile	6	Oregano	9
Camphor	5	Patchouli	5
Cardamom	9	Pennyroyal	7
Cinnamon bark	10	Peppermint	7
Clary sage	5	Petitgrain	9
Cypress	4	Rose	7
Eucalyptus	8	Rosemary	6
Fennel	6	Sandalwood	5
Frankincense	7	Spikenard	6
Geranium	6	Tea tree	6
Hyssop	6	Thyme	7
Jasmine	7	Vetiver	7
Juniper	5	Ylang ylang	6
Lavender	4		

A SIMPLE INFUSION

Lavender or rose can make a wonderful infused oil that is soothing and kind to delicate skin. Place about 2 cups (550 ml) of dried flowers or several handfuls of fresh blossoms in a large sterile jar and cover with almond or grapeseed oil. Two weeks later, strain and decant your scented oil. If you keep your infused oil cool or refrigerated, it can last for up to a year.

them, added handfuls of fresh chamomile flowers, and then filled them with almond oil. We set the jars outdoors in a warm sunny spot. After 10 days, we strained the concoction, and with luck we had a wonderfully fragrant massage oil.

I've learned a lot since those early adventures with infusion. I now know that running the jars through a hot dishwasher is also an effective means of sterilization. And I've learned the importance of drying the jars thoroughly. One drop of contaminated water at this stage can introduce bacteria, ruining your whole batch of oil. It is also a good idea to carefully blot your plants dry on paper towels or clean cotton towels. I've learned to cover the mouth of the jar with a few layers of cheesecloth and secure it with a rubber band. The cheesecloth shields the oil from insects and debris, yet allows the mixture to breathe.

In Hawaii I learned how the intensity of the tropical sun can speed up the infusion process. On my first trip to Maui I tried infusing pikake and plumeria blossoms in coconut oil. After just a few hours on the lanai, my delicate blend smelled like rotting compost. I eventually infused a wild ginger and spider lily concoction in grapeseed oil that was very good. I learned that two hours was the maximum infusion time in tropical heat, or when using very delicate tropical flowers.

FORMULARY THEORIES

Once you've mastered making an infused oil, you can experiment with different theories of how to select the ingredients for your own formulas. There are a broad range of formulary guidelines and theories to choose from, including:

Scientific method — See what others have done, study recipes in books.
Intuitive method — Use your intuitive feelings.
Astrological — Refer to the planetary influences on specific plants.
Radiesthesia — Pendulum dowsing.
Kinesiology — Muscle testing.

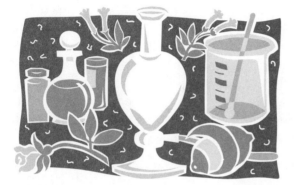

Natural
Perfumery

CHAPTER 8

The art of perfumery developed from humankind's original attempts to enhance reality through scent. Incense was probably the first means of controlled scent delivery and distribution. The word *perfume* actually means "through" *(per)* "smoke" *(fume).* Over thousands of years, perfumers' lore has passed down via oral tradition to a select few. Secrets of professional perfumery were closely guarded. Perfumers felt privileged to work with the pure essences of nature and considered their raw materials energizing and protective. It was believed in the Middle Ages that perfumers were exempt from the Plague.

An aura of mystery still permeates the world of perfume. Successful formulas are considered top secret, and perfumers jealously guard recipes and sources. Respect for the natural ingredients, however, has not remained preeminent. Sadly, most modern perfumers are trained to use synthetics, chemicals, and compounds so toxic to the nervous system that many fall ill.

THE THREE-NOTE SCALE

The classical concept of placing aromatic oils onto a three-note scale provides a structure upon which to build balanced and pleasing blends. Creating a perfume is not unlike composing a piece of music. The arrangement of a perfume resembles a three-part fugue. The part of the perfume known as the top note touches the sensibility first and vanishes in a few moments. Then the middle note, or heart, sets the theme, which can last for hours. Finally the bass note, or dry-out note, provides depth. The resonating chord of the bass note might linger for days.

Certain oils can be used as more than one note. For example, orris-root is a great fixative or bass note, but is also often used in the heart, or middle, for its soft violet scent. Angelica's rooty, animal scent makes it an effective bass note as well, while its green, acidic quality makes a good top note.

"You have to be crazy in a way," said the famous New York perfumer Sophia Grojsman about creating perfumes. "When I compose I go right to the heart of a fragrance. Some people smell top notes first. I go deeper, I search for the soul. I build my fragrance from the bottom to the top, like a pyramid, in layers. It's geometric. The art closest to what I do is music. . . . Compare your perfumes to an opera."

"You dream your perfume before you write the formula," said Jean Kerleo, a perfumer for Patou, in describing the creative process. "You begin as a composer and finish as a sculptor."

Bass Notes

Bass notes act as the foundation to a blend. Earthy, woodsy smells, they are often deep and mysterious, seductive and haunting. Bass notes are grounding to the spirit. A bass note might evoke a walk in the forest, the scent of damp humus, or an old dusty wine cellar. Without a bass note, a perfume will not last.

Some effective bass notes are:

Amber	Cistus	Mastic	Tolu balsam
Ambergris	Frankincense	Myrrh	Tonka bean
Amyris	Galbanum	Orris	Ud
Angelica	Ginger	Patchouli	Vanilla
Beeswax	Hina	Peru balsam	Vetiver
Benzoin	Labdanum	Spikenard	

Middle Notes

Middle notes are also called bouquet or heart notes. The middle note is the scent that unfolds a few moments after the application of a perfume. Herby and flowery, the middle note is like the entrée to a meal, or the stuffing in a sandwich. The middle note also has the task of weaving together the top and the bottom — just as in music, a

CLASSICAL FRAGRANCE NOTES

Note: Top
Acts upon: Spirit
Plant part: Flowers, spices

Note: Middle
Acts upon: Emotion
Plant part: Leaves, flowers

Note: Bass
Acts upon: Physical body
Plant part: Resins, wood, bark, roots

number of separate strings or notes together create a chord.

Some effective middle notes are:

Carnation	Clary sage	Petitgrain	Rosemary
Cassia	Clove bud	Pine	Tuberose
Champa	Gardenia	Orrisroot	Ylang ylang
Cinnamon	Honey	Rose	
bark	Jasmine	Rose geranium	

Top Notes

The top note is the peak, the fragrance prelude that affects the olfactory sense as a first impression. Effective top notes are delicate, light, and fresh, and are usually sweet, fruity, or spicy. They brighten up your senses and spark your attention. They are also ephemeral, leaving very quickly so you don't get too attached.

Some effective top notes are:

Artemisia	Coriander	Mandarin	Orange
Basil	Juniper	Neroli	Spice oils
Bergamot	Lavender	(orange	
Bois de rose	Lemon	blossom)	
Clary sage	Lime		

PRACTICING SCENT EVALUATION

This is really a lot of fun as well as serious work. Reserve a quiet time to work on scent evaluations. Prepare everything you will need ahead of time. Collect at least 20 or 30 different essential oils, some from each group of top, middle, and bass notes. Make perfume blotters by cutting pieces of paper into strips ⅛ inch (3 mm) wide and 6 inches (15 cm) long. Watercolor paper found in art stores works well.

Make yourself comfortable in a big soft chair with a table or desk at hand. Light a candle for inspiration. Select an oil to evaluate and write the name of the oil on one end of a paper blotter. On the other end place a drop of the oil and waft the scent by waving the blotter a few inches under your nose. Sniff lightly (avoid deep inhalations), and record your impressions on an index card. Be creative. Describe your feelings and thoughts. Imagine the scent as a color or a shape and describe it. Give it a texture. Use adjectives. You can refer to the Vocabulary of Scents on pages 161–164 for ideas.

These scent evaluation cards will become a valuable resource. Keep them for reference when you begin building perfume blends.

You may find it helpful in this process to picture an abstract perfumery color wheel. A part of the universal language of perfumery, the color wheel performs as a visual expression of scent. Imagine that the yellow-orange colors are the florals. See the hot pinks of the Oriental spices. Picture the green of the chypres, the cool mossy green of oakmoss, and the bright green of lime and bergamot.

Perfume Classifications

The International fragrance market is huge. There are more than 700 products available, including everything from feminine perfumes to classic perfumes. The H & R Genealogies is an attempt to order and categorize the perfumes on the world market similar to the classifications of styles or schools of art, such as impressionist, cubist, German expressionist, Fauvist, and so on.

Perfume styles are based on families, which in turn are subdivided into fragrance characteristics. These classifications were developed primarily from the viewpoint of the consumer. In natural perfumery, every perfume can be assessed on the basis of these fragrance styles.

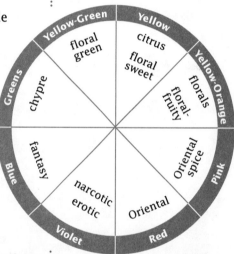

As you develop a perfume blend, it might help to think of scents in terms of corresponding colors, as indicated on this perfumery color wheel. You can select scent combinations just as you would flower colors for a perfect bouquet.

Florals. Florals are by far the most popular scents. More than half of the world's perfumes fall into this category. Floral can manifest as springlike, fresh, and light; as fruity, green, and balsamic; or in heavy floral themes.

The many branches of floral include floral green, floral fruity, floral fresh, floral floral, floral sweet, and floral aldehydic (a purely synthetic group).

Oriental. Most popular in Europe and the United States (as opposed to Asia), these woody and floral blends contain spicy ingredients like nutmeg and cinnamon. The two branches are Oriental sweet and Oriental spicy.

Chypre. Named after the island of Cyprus, all chypres (pronounced SHEE-praz) share a common theme in their bass of oakmoss, patchouli, and amber, combined with a fresh citrusy top note, usually featuring bergamot. Branches are chypre floral, chypre fresh, chypre green, chypre fruity, and chypre floral-animalic.

Fantasy. A new category of perfumes, fantasies are mostly synthetic and make no attempt to mimic the natural smells of flowers or plants. Fantasy perfumes represent an image or concept, such as "cool water" or "blue lagoon."

Study the Classics

Just as in art, music, or cooking, we can foster a familiarity with our medium by studying the work of great masters. We can learn by studying the balance and complexities of world-famous perfumes.

When using recipes and formulas, you have exact proportions or drops to follow. But experimenting with variations on classic scent themes will help you develop artistry in your blending. The following list of formulas comprises classic perfumes, along with some of my personal favorites. Since these are commercial formulas, exact combinations cannot be disclosed, but very strong oils that must be used sparingly are noted with an asterisk.

STANDARD FRAGRANCE FAMILIES

Feminine fragrance styles
1. Floral
2. Oriental
3. Chypre

Masculine fragrance styles
1. Lavender
2. Fougere
3. Oriental
4. Chypre
5. Citrus

WIND SONG BY MATCHABELLI (FLORAL FLORAL)

Top note: Bergamot, lemon, neroli, coriander*, tarragon

Middle note: Rose, clove bud*, ylang ylang*, jasmine, bois de rose

Bass note: Sandalwood, vetiver, musk, benzoin, cedar, amber, orris

WHITE SHOULDERS BY EVYAN (FLORAL FLORAL)

Top note: Neroli, green leaf, bergamot, peach, aldehydes (aldehydes are synthetics)

Middle note: Jasmine, rose, tuberose, clove*, lilac, lily-of-the-valley, orris

Bass note: Sandalwood, civet, musk, oakmoss, amber, benzoin

JICKY BY GUERLAIN (ORIENTAL SWEET)

Top note: Lemon, bergamot, mandarin, bois de rose

Middle note: Jasmine, patchouli, rose, orris, vetiver

Bass note: Vanilla, benzoin, amber, tonka, civet, frankincense, leather

4711 BY MULHENS (CITRUS FRESH)

Top note: Bergamot, lemon, orange, petitgrain, neroli*

Middle note: Rosemary, rose

Bass note: Musk (musk substitutes are amber, ambrette seed, angelica*)

PARIS BY YVES ST.-LAURENT (FLORAL FLORAL)

Top note: Green notes, bergamot, hyacinth, calyx

Middle note: Violet, Damascena rose, orris, jasmine, linden

Bass note: Musk, cedarwood, oakmoss, sandalwood, heliotrope

MILLE = 1000 BY PATOU (FLORAL FLORAL)

Top note: Green notes, bergamot, coriander, tarragon, angelica

Middle note: Rose, geranium, lily-of-the-valley, orris, jasmine

Bass note: Patchouli, vetiver, oakmoss, sandalwood, musk, amber, civet

GIORGIO BY GIORGIO BEVERLY HILLS (FLORAL FLORAL)

Top note: Green notes, bergamot, fruit note, orange blossom, aldehydes (synthetics)

Middle note: Tuberose, gardenia, jasmine, ylang ylang, orchid

Bass note: Sandalwood, cedarwood, musk, amber, oakmoss, vanilla

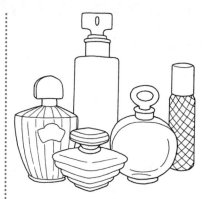

One of the best ways to train your nose to be sensitive to the subtleties of scent is to study the classic perfumes and try to identify the elements hidden within.

CHLOE BY KARL LAGERFELD (FLORAL FLORAL)
Top note: Green notes, coconut, bergamot, aldehydes (synthetics), peach
Middle note: Tuberose, jasmine, ylang ylang, hyacinth, orris
Bass note: Musk, sandalwood, oakmoss, amber, cedar, benzoin

CHARLIE BY REVLON (FLORAL FLORAL)
Top note: Citrus, peach, hyacinth, tarragon
Middle note: Jasmine, rose, lily-of-the-valley, cyclamen, carnation, orris
Bass note: Cedarwood, sandalwood, oakmoss, musk, vanilla

YOUTH DEW BY ESTEE LAUDER (ORIENTAL SPICY)
Top note: Orange, spice, bergamot, peach
Middle note: Carnation, rose, ylang ylang, cassia, cinnamon, jasmine
Bass note: Amber, tolu, patchouli, frankincense, oakmoss, Peru balsam, benzoin, vanilla

SHALIMAR BY GUERLAIN (ORIENTAL SWEET)
Top note: Lemon, bergamot, mandarin, bois de rose
Middle note: Patchouli, rose, jasmine, orris, vetiver
Bass note: Opopanax, vanilla, benzoin, Peru balsam, leather (birch resin)

JOY BY PATOU (FLORAL FLORAL)
Top note: Leafy green, peach, flower notes
Middle note: Rose, jasmine, ylang ylang, orris, orchid, muguet (French for lily-of-the-valley)
Bass note: Sandalwood, musk (musk substitutes are amber and ambrette seed), civet, angelica root

CANOE BY DANA (FLORAL SWEET)
Top note: Lavender, clary sage, lemon
Middle note: Geranium, carnation, cedarwood, patchouli
Bass note: Vanilla, tonka, musk (musk substitutes are amber, ambrette seed, and angelica root), heliotrope, oakmoss

Clear Your Olfactory Palate

When you work with different scents, it is important to clear your olfactory palate. Just as wine tasters use white bread or crackers to clear their palates between tasting different wines, or sushi eaters take a bit of *gari* (pickled ginger) between tasting different types of fish, perfumers must clear their olfactory palates to keep their sense of smell tuned.

I keep a small piece of wool or a 100 percent wool scarf close at hand whenever I work with scents in a creative way. At regular intervals I hold the fabric over my nose and mouth and take a few breaths. The wool effectively filters the air and cleanses the palate, preparing the nasal passage for optimum appreciation of the next scent. A small piece of natural sea salt on the tongue can have a similar effect. I prefer the chunky type of sea salt, although this can be hard to find. Some perfumers clear their palates by sniffing fresh coffee beans. All of these methods work. I recommend you experiment with each method and choose the one that seems to work best for you.

When working with scents, always be sure to step outside for a breath of fresh air every hour or so. The fresh air will clear your head, renew your creativity, and preserve your scent acuity.

Keep a Notebook or Card File

Always take notes when experimenting with your oils. I use a card file and keep my formulas written on index cards; you can also enter notes on a computer later (away from the oils), if desired. Use the same recipe format so you can compare the middle, top, and bass notes easily. It is tragic to create a beautiful blend and not remember how you did it. Each drop makes a difference.

On page 156 is a sample card. On it, you'd record the name of each oil you use in a formula, along with the exact number of drops. A typical proportion is 30 ml (1 ounce) perfume alcohol and 100 drops of essential oils.

Using this or a similar format, you can perform a laboratory experiment or create a spontaneous work of art. You will find what feels most comfortable for you and develop your own unique style.

Blend name: _____

Date developed: _____

Top note: _____

Middle note: _____

Bass note: _____

Comments: _____

_____

_____

FORMULAS FOR BUILDING BLENDS

There are "formulas" to perfumery just as there are "formulas" to music, fine cuisine, and the arts. Certain combinations just work: In music a repeat phrase or a return to the chorus line makes a melody pleasing to the ear; in visual art, analogous color schemes please the eye. Sometimes art is shocking or dramatic, and there is also a formula for that.

Study similarities in top, middle, and bass notes. Look at the common denominators. As you become familiar with the formulas, you will begin to understand the language of scent used by perfumers for hundreds of years.

I always begin with bass notes and combine 3 to 10 different substances. If the blend lasts on a blotter for more than three days, I consider it a good fixative. A rule of thumb is that the bass should never equal more than 20 percent of the total.

Think about your favorite perfumes. What are some of the qualities of perfumes you like? Are they sweet? Are they light and fresh or deep and amberlike? Do you want your creation to be sweet? green? fresh? ancient? rich? musty?

This is a creative place. Let your mind, your emotions, your imagination, and your memory all work together here. Some perfumers listen to inspirational music as they "compose" a new scent.

To conduct the following experiments prepare all your equipment and ingredients and create some quiet, uninterrupted time.

A Perfume-Blending Experiment

To begin your blending, you will need to assemble the following:

Equipment and Materials

- 120 ml (4-ounce) glass beaker or jar
- Clean hand towel or paper towels
- Wooden chopsticks or glass straw
- Coffee filters
- Perfumer's alcohol
- Distilled or floral water
- Essential oils
- Flacon for finished perfume
- Prepared perfume-formula index cards

Most of the equipment needed for blending perfumes can be found right in your own kitchen. You might want to reuse old perfume bottles or search antique shops for unusual ones to fit your blend.

For this perfume, use standard proportions: 70 percent alcohol base, 20 percent water, and 10 percent essential oils.

1. Choose one of the formulas from the list of classic perfumes and select the top, middle, and bass notes you will use. Remember to record your formula on a prepared index card.

2. Start with 90 ml (3 ounces) of a high-quality perfumer's alcohol. Although some perfumers recommend ethyl or grain alcohol, and even vodka, I find that a high-quality perfumer's alcohol (wine alcohol) gives much finer results.

3. Add your notes, beginning with the bass. If you need help determining proportions of oils within notes, refer to the Odor Intensity Guide on page 145. Shake to mix after the introduction of each oil.

4. Finally, add distilled water or hydrosol very sparingly. Too much water can turn your perfume cloudy. To remedy this you can either add more alcohol or filter your perfume through a coffee filter and then chill it in the freezer for an hour or so.

Alcohol- or Oil-Based Perfumes?

The commercially marketed fragrance products we know as perfumes are usually a mix of aromatic oils in a 75 to 95 percent alcohol solution. Real perfume, the finest and most expensive of these products, has a concentration of aromatic oils greater than 22 percent. Eau de perfume has a 15 to 22 percent concentration, and eau de toilette has an 8 to 15 percent concentration. The most diluted is cologne, which contains less than 5 percent aromatic oils, and some water.

For commercial purposes, extending the essences in alcohol is cost effective, but you can create your own custom blends with or without alcohol. Some fine perfumeries use only essential oils, adding no alcohol or other diluents. Others feel that pure essences are too strong to be enjoyed properly and must be diluted in alcohol.

Oil-based perfumes dating back to ancient Egypt are gaining in popularity. The main advantage of oil-based perfumes is you can melt beeswax into them for a solid balm, or add the oil-based perfume to creams, body oils, or bath salts.

The disadvantage of oil-based perfumes is the necessity of heating solids and resins to blend, as opposed to the easier solvent reaction response of alcohol-based perfumes.

BUILDING YOUR PERFUME FROM THE BOTTOM UP

To build your perfume from the bottom up you will begin with your bass notes, which should amount to no more than 20 percent of the total formula. Sixty percent of the formula should be built from middle notes, and the remaining 20 percent or so will be the top notes.

Make an Oil-Based Perfume

For this perfume you will use jojoba oil as your base or carrier oil.

Equipment and Materials

- Small enamel or glass saucepan
- 120 ml (4-ounce) glass beaker or jar
- Clean hand towel or paper towels
- Wooden chopsticks
- Jojoba oil
- Aromatic oils
- Prepared perfume-formula index cards

1. Measure 30 ml (1 ounce) of jojoba into the glass beaker or jar.

2. Select your bass notes and add a total of 20 to 30 drops to the jojoba oil in the beaker. If you are using solids or thick resins such as vanilla in your bass, you will have to guess at your measurements, and you will need to melt them in the jojoba. To do this, place the beaker in the saucepan filled halfway with water. Heat over a medium flame, stirring constantly with a wooden chopstick until the resins are melted into the jojoba. Do not use metal utensils, which may interact negatively with your oils.

3. Remove from the heat and add a total of 60 to 90 drops of middle notes. Choose four to six from the list, shaking or stirring after you add each oil. Finally, add your top notes, in roughly equal proportion to the bass notes. Decant your perfume into an attractive glass bottle with a tight-fitting lid. Allow the blend a few days to "marry." A well-balanced blend will not have jagged edges or strikingly dominant scents.

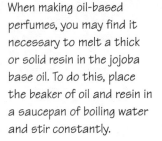

When making oil-based perfumes, you may find it necessary to melt a thick or solid resin in the jojoba base oil. To do this, place the beaker of oil and resin in a saucepan of boiling water and stir constantly.

Make a Salve or Solid Perfume

Solid perfumes or unguents are easy to create by just adding a little melted beeswax to the liquid perfume.

Equipment and Materials

- 2 small enamel or glass saucepans
- 120 ml (4 ounce) glass beaker or jar
- Clean hand towel or paper towels
- Wooden chopsticks
- Coffee filters
- Beeswax
- Jojoba oil
- Aromatic oils
- Prepared perfume-formula index cards

Determine proportions using this formula: 100 drops of essential oil to 30 ml (1 ounce) of carrier or base. The base will consist of 1 part beeswax to 4 parts jojoba for a slightly hard, solid product. For a softer solid, adjust the proportion to 1 part beeswax to 5 parts jojoba.

1. Choose your top, middle, and bass notes, and remember to record the final proportions on an index card.

2. Melt the beeswax in one saucepan over low heat, stirring with a chopstick. Gently heat the jojoba oil by placing it in the glass beaker in the other saucepan, filled halfway with water. Mix the warmed jojoba with the hot beeswax. If there is any sediment in this beeswax-jojoba mixture, filter it through cheesecloth or a coffee filter while still liquid.

3. Immediately pour the hot wax-and-oil mixture into a clean jar, add your essential oils, and stir. Work quickly at this point in order to thoroughly blend your perfume before it begins to solidify.

4. Cover and allow the mixture to set for about 20 minutes. To test for hardness you can place the jar in the freezer for 5 to 10 minutes before checking. For a nice smooth surface, it is important not to disturb the jar while it sets up.

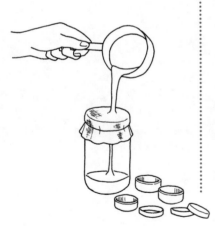

If you're making solid perfume, strain the melted beeswax-jojoba mixture through a piece of cheesecloth to filter out any sediment.

THE VOCABULARY OF SCENTS

In 1988 I attended "Future Scents," an aromatherapy conference in northern California. One of the lecturers was John Steele, an enthusiastic scholar of archaeology, anthropology, and geology. John spoke of our language's lack of vocabulary to describe scent. He pointed out how a more descriptive language could help us to better communicate about odors and describe more eloquently what our noses are sensing. I thought this was a fabulous idea, and started working on this new vocabulary right away.

I have been collecting a growing dictionary of scent terms and here share what I have compiled so far. Some of these words are "borrowed" from vintner's terminology; many are adapted from French, the language with the most extensive scent vocabulary. Many of these words express abstract perceptions. Adding some of them to your vocabulary will enable you to express more fully what your nose communicates to you.

Accord. A balanced complex of three or four notes that lose their individuality to create a completely new, unified odor impression.

Adaptation. A tolerance to a particular perfume or scent so that it becomes unrecognizable.

Alcohol. Smelling of rubbing or ethyl alcohol.

Aldehyde. A synthetic scent with a rich opulence; a recognizable top note with a lemony or lemongrass scent.

Animal note. A sensual, heady bass note associated with the animal source oils: musk, civet, ambergris, and castoreum. Smelling of fecal odors. Animal notes can also be achieved from vegetable sources such as angelica, cistus, ambrette, and jasmine.

Anisic. Having a licorice-like odor of aniseed or fennel.

Balsamic. Having the sweet, soft, warm odor of resins.

Bass note. This is the bottom note and may show great tenacity. It acts as a fixative. Also called the dry-out note, it may occur only after several hours, and may continue for several days.

Blue. A scent in nature that is very elusive and hard to capture. Blue smells synthetic: total fantasy, as cool blue, blue water, rain, blue sky, dry seaweed scent.

Boeuf. A bad smell, like rotten meat (from the French word for "beef").

Bouquet. A subtle, well-balanced blend of two or more fragrances. In French, the term refers to the combined floral quality of a smell.

Camphorous. Smelling of camphor, like mothballs.

Chypre. Pronounced SHEE-pra. A fragrance blend described as heavy and clinging with a flowery characteristic. A fruity eau de Cologne with an oakmoss bass.

Citrus. The fresh tangy smell of lemon, lime, orange, and so on. Citrus smells are considered antierogenous.

Cool. A term to describe outdoorsy scents such as green leaves after a rain, bracing mint notes, and citrus.

Cush. A funky still smell of residue from the last distillation; a sulfur smell.

Diffusion. A spontaneous vibrancy that causes a fragrance to radiate around your being.

Dry. A term to describe a fragrance that lacks sweetness, for instance one with woody notes.

Dry-out note. The residual odor left after the volatile components have evaporated.

Earthy. The aroma of freshly turned soil. The scent is achieved with oakmoss, patchouli and vetiver, or spikenard.

Erlenmeyer flask. A laboratory glass (aka vas de Florentine) used to catch the finished distillation of water and oil.

Essential oil. Essence; etheric oil; volatile oil.

Evaluate. In perfume testing, short little sniffs rather than long, deep inhalations are used for evaluation.

Factice. An oversize display perfume flacon (bottle); it holds tinted liquid.

Fixative. Derived from resins, mosses, and roots, fixatives modify the evaporation rate of a perfume's note-giving element and make the scent lasting.

Florentine vase. Also called a Florence container and Erlenmeyer flask, a container used in the distillation process to catch the completed distillation of water and oil.

Foresty. Resembling the odor of wood, or the woods.

Fresh. A brisk, lively character of citrus or green composition.

Fruity. Any of the sweet fruit smells, such as apple and orange.

Green. A grasslike scent: dry, clean, and bright.

Herbaceous. Having an odor of herbs and garden plants (from the Greek *forbea,* meaning "pasture").

Jagged edges. Prominent notes; failure to blend; lacking synergy.

Ketones. Jagged, powerful, medicinal, sharp, and abrasive.

Leather. Musky odor with a distinct smell of animal hides.

Marriage. The interval of time that ensures proper blending. For a fragrance to blend properly, it needs a few days to "marry" or "age."

Mellow. A fragrance that has achieved a perfect balance; a smooth, rich fragrance.

Metallic. Having a cool, clear effect, like a steel pan after it's rinsed with cool water.

Middle note. This is the bouquet or heart note composed of leaves and flowers; it may occur for two to three hours.

Mossy. Earthy, green, humus smelling.

Mousy. Not a good smell; a bit animal-like.

Note. A single impression in fragrance; a vibration.

Oriental spice. A classification of perfumes with a common theme of amber-patchouli-vanilla in the bass note, and cinnamon and spices on top.

Peppery. Hot and spicy; exotic. Scents of black or green pepper.

Pot odor. In French, *vegetalle.* A sulfury odor present in an essential oil or floral water immediately upon distillation.

COLORS FROM NATURE

Pick red rose petals and place them in a bottle of pure alcohol. When the alcohol has absorbed the rose color, hold or "fix" it by placing the container of alcohol in the freezer for a few hours. Use the colored alcohol to color a perfume. Experiment with other colors. Wilted petals of purple iris make a lovely robin's egg blue. Violet flowers of wisteria make lavender, and pomegranate seeds yield a violet-fuchsia.

Powdery. Having a rather indistinct odor. A certain blend of florals similar to the smell of baby's powder or a baby's head attains this highly desirable smell.

Pungent. Piercing and spicy; a smell with a hot character similar to pepper.

Refined. Having an exquisite quality. Pursuing perfection.

Relaxing. Calming and soothing to the emotions.

Rich. Full, with intensified depth and harmony.

Rose scent of Mary. A religious idea of what Mary's natural scent is.

Round. Perfectly toned and complete in effect.

Scent of sanctity. A saint's natural bodily emanations, or those of a spiritually evolved being.

Sharp. A peak or certain blend that is too strong; needs softening.

Sniffing. The act of inhaling in short little drafts to get the effects of an odor. See *evaluate.*

Soft. A very light, innocent effect; bois de rose is an example.

Tropical fruit. A difficult-to-achieve scent that blends oils, fruits, and flowers of Indian origin: specifically kewda and champa oils.

Warm. An aroma with a rich, heating action.

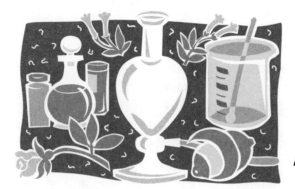

Aphrodisiacs

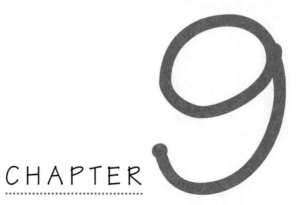

CHAPTER 9

Throughout history mankind has traveled the scented path in pursuit of romance. Romance is what distinguishes human sexual activity from the mating behavior of lower animals. Romance is about love and beauty and the sharing of pleasure. Romance is atmosphere and fantasy, magic and illusion, and ultimately romance is about sex.

The Scent of a Loved One

The smell that we first react to in a person transmits a wealth of information on a cellular level. When we say there is "chemistry" between two people, we are describing an invisible connection that is felt at an emotional level.

Just as hormones are secreted within our bodies, pheromones are secreted into our environment. Like hormones, pheromones are chemical messengers that are only just beginning to be understood. We do know that pheromones are scent signals sent by one animal to another of the opposite sex, in the same species. The word is a combination of the Greek words *pherein* (to bear along) and *hormon* (an excitement).

We know the effect of a pheromone between insects is compelling. Although pheromones do not necessarily work in the same way with humans, links between sex and scent are certainly present. Smell is a good indicator of health. Our sense of smell influences our ability to produce hormones. Studies indicate that one-quarter of those people who lose their sense of smell suffer from diminished libidos.

Every individual has a unique odor to his or her skin. Apocrine glands, modified sebaceous glands clustered on the face, under the arms, on the chest, and in the genital areas, produce a distinct individualized scent. This scent mixes with the sweat, flora, and bacteria on the surface of our skin, along with any scent we add intentionally, to create every individual's unique odor. This individual chemistry is why the same scent will smell differently on different people.

Women are most sensitive to smell during periods of peak fertility. It is during this time also that a woman's scent becomes stronger and most agreeable to men. In reaction, the male produces odor to the degree of his arousal, which in turn sends a message to the woman. These complex communications take place so subtly that we remain largely unaware of them. Although we spend a lot of effort in disguising our natural odors, they probably influence our sexual attraction and bonding more than all the perfumes, deodorants, and aftershaves that we so carefully select.

Creating Romance with Aroma

I like to create a sensual atmosphere using scented oils and fresh flowers, soft music and candlelight, bubble baths, champagne, and sensual foods like chocolate or oysters.

My favorite aphrodisiac oils are cinnamon, sandalwood, clary sage, tonka, jasmine, tuberose, narcissus, vanilla, patchouli, ylang ylang, and rose.

Other oils considered sexually stimulating include ambrette, mace, angelica, neroli, basil, nutmeg, bois de rose, peppermint, clove, pine, cumin, sage, fennel, savory, ginger, thyme, and juniper.

"SCENTUAL" BATHING

Bathing together in itself can be a sensual, bonding ritual. A shared bath provides the opportunity for partners to pamper each other in a tactile and nurturing fashion. In the seclusion of the bath, you can explore your partner's body and experiment with sensual touch.

Essential oils, used alone or in combination, along with soft lights, special soaps, and oversize sponges or loofahs can turn a simple cleansing routine into a romantic affair. Add the oils after the bath is filled. The oils will float on the surface of the water, dispersing as you enter the bath.

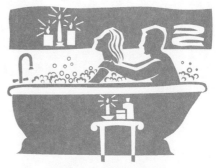

Try combinations of three of the aphrodisiac oils listed on page 167. Start with four or five drops of each oil mixed together in a cup (235 ml) of milk.

Bath salts will mineralize and increase the buoyancy of your bath. You can make scented bath salts by sprinkling a total of about 60 drops (3 ml) over 4 cups (1,100 ml) of Epsom salts. Add a few drops of food color if you want a colored bath. Stir the salts to mix the oil and color and store in a sealed quart-size (l) jar. Allow a few days for the oils to permeate the salts. Add ½ to 1 cup (140 to 275 ml) of these scented salts as the bath is filling.

WINTER WARMING BATH

Both of these blends are warming and stimulating, the perfect choice for an invigorating soak before climbing into bed with your partner on a cold, foggy evening.

Formula 1

    4   drops savory essential oil
    4   drops ginger essential oil
    4   drops juniper essential oil
  235   ml (1 cup) milk

Formula 2

    4   drops sandalwood essential oil
    4   drops myrrh essential oil
    4   drops ginger essential oil
  235   ml (1 cup) milk

Stir the essential oils into the milk and mix well.
To use: Disperse blend in the bath.

Avant L'Amour Bath Blend

4 drops jasmine essential oil
4 drops ginger essential oil
2 drops cumin essential oil
4 drops neroli essential oil
6 drops clary sage essential oil
235 ml (1 cup) milk

Stir the essential oils into the milk and mix well.
To use: Disperse blend in the bath.

THE LOVING TOUCH

Touch is one of our most primitive and potent forms of communication. Giving or receiving a massage, enhanced with the appropriate aromas, can work wonders in opening the gates of reserve and releasing repressed sensuality.

Experiment with the oils listed for their aphrodisiac qualities. You can select one oil for its scent or combine up to three or four with a carrier oil of your choice. A total of 20 to 30 drops of essential oil to 1 ounce (30 ml) of carrier oil is a good ratio to begin experimenting with. Note that sage and thyme should be avoided by anyone with elevated blood pressure, and fennel should be avoided by anyone subject to seizures. Cinnamon and ginger are very stimulating and warming oils, and should only be used on the skin in a highly diluted form. For safety, use no more than 4 drops of cinnamon or ginger to 1 ounce (30 ml) of carrier oil for massage purposes.

There are many excellent books on massage technique. Basically you will need quiet and privacy in a warm room with a comfortably firm surface. Massage oil, besides being the vehicle of delivery for the aroma, serves as a lubricant, decreasing friction and allowing the long, slow, smooth strokes that are so soothing to the body and spirit.

Valentine Blend

Surprise your lover on Valentine's Day with this yummy oil. Start the evening by sharing a sensual massage and let your imagination lead you down pleasure's path.

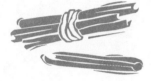

  60 ml (2 ounces) glycerin
  60 ml (2 ounces) almond oil
    2 drops cinnamon essential oil
    2 drops peppermint essential oil
    3 ml (¾ teaspoon) beet juice

Mix the glycerin and almond oil in a 120 ml (4 ounce) glass bottle. Add the cinnamon and peppermint essential oils and the beet juice to make a mild, safe, edible body oil blend.

Eros and Psyche's Perfumed Body Oil

To make a massage oil using this formula, increase the carrier oil to 2 ounces (60 ml) and decrease the essential oils by half.

  20 drops cinnamon essential oil
  40 drops myrrh essential oil
  60 drops patchouli essential oil
  40 drops clove essential oil
   5 ml (1 teaspoon) bois de rose essential oil
  40 drops rose essential oil
  60 ml (2 ounces) carrier oil

Blend the essential oils with the carrier oil of your choice in a 120 ml (4 ounce) dark glass bottle and shake to mix.
To use: This blend will make a sensuous perfumed body oil. A few drops applied to the torso, lower back, or inner thigh area will

enhance a sensual mood. This blend should not be applied directly to the genital area or around the eyes, because the cinnamon is irritating to mucous membranes and delicate skin.

SCENTUAL BODY POWDER

Scented body powders are easy to make and a wonderful way of pampering yourself or your lover.

> 60 g (2 ounces) white clay
> 2 drops petitgrain essential oil
> 2 drops neroli essential oil
> 4 drops sandalwood essential oil

Mix the white clay powder with the essential oils in a widemouthed jar with a tight-fitting lid and blend well.

To use: Dust each other with a big soft puff after sharing a bath, or try a massage with powder instead of a massage oil. The silky texture will decrease friction nearly as effectively as an oil and leave you feeling warm, dry, and softly scented.

APRÉS L'AMOUR

The tremendous sense of peace and well-being that descends after orgasm is an important facet of physical love. For a brief period we are lulled by the ultimate intimacy, and we experience a profound connection to our lover. Rather than turning over and falling off to sleep, savor these blissful moments by prolonging skin-to-skin contact. According to ancient Taoist tradition, aprés l'amour is an especially alchemical time. If the penis is allowed to rest in, or close to, the vagina after lovemaking, a wonderful exchange of male-female energies occurs. These formulas were created to enhance this special time.

ROMANCE YOUR INNER MATE

People naturally experience different degrees of sexuality at different times in their lives. Can you be romantic by yourself? We all must love ourselves before we can truly accept the love of another. We will all find ourselves alone at some point in our lives. Learn how to cherish yourself and become the beloved of your lover.

AFTERGLOW BLEND

Formula 1

 5 drops ylang ylang essential oil

 5 drops tonka essential oil

 5 drops palmarosa essential oil

 5 drops nutmeg essential oil

Formula 2

 5 drops jasmine essential oil

 5 drops frankincense essential oil

 5 drops sandalwood essential oil

Formula 3

 5 drops cardamom essential oil

 5 drops jasmine essential oil

 5 drops rose essential oil

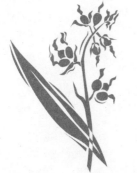

Blend oils in a small glass vial with a tight-fitting stopper and mix well.
To use: It may take some special planning and logistics to use these blends in the true spirit of Taoism. Keep a small vial close at hand for inhalation following lovemaking. Or prepare a drop or two on a cotton ball, place it in a lidded glass dish next to the bed, and when the moment is right, remove the lid. A diffuser can also be prepared ahead. Or mix the oils with an ounce (30 ml) of distilled water in a small sprayer to mist. The blends can also be mixed with an ounce of carrier oil for a powerful aprés l'amour massage.

AROMATHERAPY AND SEXUAL DYSFUNCTION

Stress, anxiety, and depression are probably the leading causes of sexual malaise in our modern culture. Sexual dysfunction can also result from organic disorders, or disease and its resulting treatments.

Once these factors have been ruled out or dealt with medically, getting back on track can be merely a matter of achieving balance in the nervous system, the endocrine system, or the emotional system.

Although testosterone is considered the male hormone, it is also produced (in smaller measure) in the female system. The presence of testosterone is crucial to a lusty libido. Neither a man nor a woman is likely to be interested in sex without sufficient testosterone. The hormone-balancing properties of specific essential oils are of particular value in such cases.

A natural sex drive is a measure of good health. The autonomic nervous system is the part of the nervous system that is responsible for control and regulation of involuntary bodily functions, including those of the heart, circulatory system, and glandular activity. It consists of the sympathetic nervous system, which stimulates the body to prepare for physical action or emergency, and the parasympathetic, which in general stimulates the opposite responses. Sexual arousal and orgasm are achieved through a delicate interplay of these two systems. The parasympathetic system dominates during arousal. As the intensity of the encounter builds, the sympathetic system takes over, flooding the bloodstream with adrenaline until orgasm takes place. If the sympathetic and parasympathetic systems are not working in synchronicity, sexual dysfunction can be a primary symptom. Premature ejaculation in men and difficulty in achieving orgasm in women are often signs of an imbalance in the autonomic nervous system.

In olfactory studies conducted at Toho University in Japan, Professor Shizuo Torii has demonstrated the influence of specific essential oils on the sympathetic branch of the autonomic nervous system. These oils include jasmine, ylang ylang, rose, patchouli, peppermint, neroli, clove, bois de rose, and basil. Torii also found that the action of the parasympathetic nervous system was increased by sandalwood, marjoram, lemon, chamomile, and bergamot. Professor Torii's findings represent the first scientific validation of the use of specific essential oils to treat sexual dysfunction.

Male Hormonal Balancing Blend

For a man who is experiencing premature ejaculation, Torii's studies would indicate the use of oils in support of the parasympathetic nervous system. Massage with the following blend would support the male hormonal system and be a balancing influence to the autonomic nervous system.

> 10 drops bergamot essential oil
> 2 drops chamomile essential oil
> 6 drops sandalwood essential oil
> 3 drops lemon essential oil
> 60 ml (2 ounces) apricot oil

Mix all ingredients in a 60 ml (2 ounce) bottle and shake well.

Female Hormonal Balancing Blend

For a woman who is experiencing difficulty in achieving orgasm, Torii's studies would indicate the use of oils in support of the sympathetic nervous system. Massage with the following blend would support the female hormonal system and be a balancing influence to the autonomic nervous system.

> 10 drops ylang ylang essential oil
> 2 drops jasmine essential oil
> 3 drops patchouli essential oil
> 3 drops clove essential oil
> 3 drops geranium essential oil
> 60 ml (2 ounces) apricot oil

Mix all ingredients in a 60 ml (2 ounce) bottle and shake well.

Breast-Enhancing Formula

Formula 1

   10 drops fennel essential oil
   10 drops clary sage essential oil
   10 drops geranium essential oil
   30 ml (1 ounce) almond oil

Formula 2

    5 drops angelica essential oil
    5 drops lemongrass essential oil
   10 drops cypress essential oil
   30 ml (1 ounce) almond oil

Combine all ingredients in a small dark glass bottle and shake well to blend.

To use: Massage onto your chest area daily. The hormonal properties of the ingredient oils will improve skin texture and plump up underlying tissue to give your breasts a more youthful appearance. Better yet, let your husband or lover apply the oils. You will no doubt discover that he is enthralled with your breasts just as they are, and you will both benefit from the tactile stimulation and from your renewed body confidence.

LOVEMAKING SUPPORT

If you or your partner are both "in the mood" but the mechanics aren't working properly you might try one of the following formulas.

BODY CONFIDENCE

It has been said that our most important sex organ is the brain, and the most important sexual stimulant is our emotions. If we are distracted by stressful circumstances in our lives, we may not enjoy lovemaking. We may not even think about sex, or we may be unable to keep our thoughts focused during a sexual interlude.

Body consciousness has an enormous influence on our sexual response. Women tend to be self-conscious about their bodies, focusing on their imperfections. This self-consciousness can be so distracting that it interferes with their pleasure in sex. These two formulas can boost your confidence if you feel inadequate about the size or texture of your breasts.

Male Support Blend

Erection problems can be simply a result of poor circulation in the genital area.

  4 drops anise vert (green seed) essential oil
  5 drops basil essential oil
  4 drops clove essential oil
  5 drops ginger essential oil
 60 ml (2 ounces) carrier oil

Combine the essential oils with the carrier oil of your choice in a 60 ml (2 ounce) dark glass bottle and shake to mix.

To use: Massage onto perineum points between anus and testicles to stimulate circulation and support healthy erectile function.

Warming Up Blend

If frigidity or impotence is an issue, try this warming bath blend.

  4 drops angelica essential oil
  4 drops black pepper essential oil
  2 drops cinnamon essential oil
 10 drops bois de rose essential oil
235 ml (1 cup) milk or solubol

Stir the essential oils into the milk or solubol and mix well.

To use: Disperse in a comfortably warm bath. Soak for at least 20 minutes, adding hot water as needed to maintain temperature.

LOVE POTIONS

Whether or not you believe in the magic of love potions, essential oils do have the power to leave an indelible impression on a lover's mind. When the initial heady stages of romantic love are associated with a unique scent, that scent becomes imprinted on the brain. Years later, long after the "bloom has faded from the vine," the slightest whiff of that same scent can trigger the scent memory, and evoke the emotions of a love lost to the distant past.

Love spells have always played a prominent role in legend and myth. With their power to influence memory, emotion, and physiology, it's no wonder that essential oils are a traditional ingredient in potions to influence love. If you are inclined to test the magic of essential oils, try a few of these formulas.

ISOLDE AND TRISTAN'S BINDING LOVE BLEND

This potion is named for the doomed lovers who were bound for life after sharing a magic love elixir.

    20 drops champa essential oil
    20 drops tuberose essential oil
    80 drops ylang ylang essential oil
    40 drops jasmine essential oil
    22 ml (1½ tablespoons) white wine

Combine all ingredients in a 30 ml (1 ounce) bottle and shake to mix.

To use: Add a few drops of this blend to a glass of champagne and share it with your lover to bind your hearts for eternity (see caution regarding internal use on page 131). A few drops placed over the heart will have the same effect.

ARIANNE'S BLEND

Use this pulse-point balm when love is struggling to survive. Apply a small amount to the pulse points at the inner wrists, behind the knees, and along the hairline at the back of the neck.

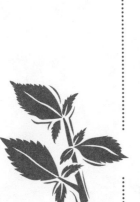

 5 g (²/₁₀ ounce) beeswax
 5 ml (1 teaspoon) jojoba oil
 5 ml (1 teaspoon) bois de rose essential oil
 5 ml (1 teaspoon) orange essential oil
 3 ml (³/₄ teaspoon) lime essential oil
40 drops vetiver essential oil
40 drops myrrh essential oil
 5 ml (1 teaspoon) cedar essential oil
40 drops frankincense essential oil
20 drops everlasting essential oil

1. Melt the beeswax in a small saucepan over low heat, stirring with a wooden chopstick.

2. Gently heat the jojoba oil by placing it in a glass beaker in another saucepan filled halfway with water.

3. Mix the warmed jojoba with the hot beeswax. If there is any sediment in this beeswax-jojoba mixture, you can clear it by pouring it through cheesecloth or a coffee filter while it is still liquid.

4. Immediately pour the hot wax-and-oil mixture into a clean jar, add essential oils, and stir. You will need to work quickly at this point in order to thoroughly blend your balm before it begins to solidify.

5. Cover and allow the mixture to set for about 20 minutes. For a nice smooth surface, it is important not to disturb the balm while it is setting up.

BLEND TO ATTRACT LOVE

 5 drops cardamom essential oil
15 drops palmarosa essential oil
 5 drops rose essential oil
30 ml (1 ounce) jojoba oil

Combine oils in a 30 ml (1 ounce) dark glass bottle. Shake to mix.
To use: Apply to the pulse points at the inner wrists, behind the knees, and along the hairline at the back of the neck.

BLEND TO BRING A LOVER BACK

 5 drops honeysuckle absolute
 5 drops carnation absolute
 5 drops tuberose essential oil
30 ml (1 ounce) jojoba oil

Combine ingredients in a 30 ml (1 ounce) dark glass bottle. Shake to mix.
To use: Apply to the pulse points at the inner wrists, behind the knees, and along the hairline at the back of the neck.

BLEND TO STIMULATE EROTIC LONGING

10 drops jasmine essential oil
10 drops rose essential oil
10 drops ylang ylang essential oil
30 ml (1 ounce) jojoba oil

Combine oils in a 30 ml (1 ounce) dark glass bottle. Shake to mix.
To use: Apply to the pulse points at the inner wrists, behind the knees, and along the hairline at the back of the neck.

IN YOUR DREAMS

If you are wishing for a new love to come into your life, you might try dreaming of your future love. A few drops of either neroli and sandalwood, or mimosa, rubbed into your forehead before going to sleep can stimulate prophetic dreams. You can also mix the same oils into a spray bottle with 1 ounce (30 ml) of hydrosol or distilled water. Shake well and mist your pillows with it.

Smelling mugwort before retiring will enhance your ability to recall your dreams. I like to cut fresh mugwort and hang it to dry it in my bedroom.

BLEND TO HEAL A REJECTED HEART

20 drops lavender essential oil   5 drops geranium essential oil
5 drops patchouli essential oil   2 drops jasmine essential oil
10 drops bergamot essential oil   60 ml (2 ounces) carrier oil

Combine the essential oils with a carrier oil of your choice in a 60 ml (2 ounce) dark glass bottle and shake to mix.

To use: Apply to the pulse points at the inner wrists, behind the knees, and along the hairline at the back of the neck.

BLEND TO RECOVER FROM LOSS OF A LOVED ONE

12 drops ud essential oil
12 drops rose essential oil
30 ml (1 ounce) jojoba oil

Combine oils in a 30 ml (1 ounce) dark glass bottle. Shake to mix.

To use: Anoint the heart area and the forehead.

BLEND TO ASSUAGE GRIEF OVER A RELATIONSHIP

5 drops rose essential oil
5 drops neroli essential oil
15 drops cedarwood essential oil
5 drops spikenard essential oil
30 ml (1 ounce) jojoba oil

Combine oils in a 30 ml (1 ounce) dark glass bottle. Shake to mix.

To use: Apply to the pulse points at the inner wrists, behind the knees, and along the hairline at the back of the neck.

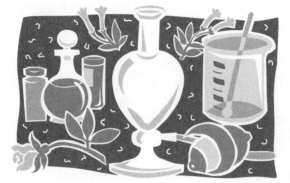

Aromatherapy
and Ayurveda

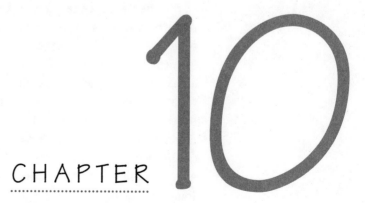

CHAPTER 10

Ayurveda is the oldest system of medicine in the world. Deeply spiritual in origin, it is the base from which most other medical systems have sprung. Ayurvedic works were translated into Chinese around A.D. 400 and exerted great influence on Chinese medicine and herbology. Several hundred years later, with Arabic translations, Ayurvedic principles were influencing Islamic medicine. In the 16th century, Paracelsus, a Swiss-born alchemist and physician, borrowed heavily from Ayurveda to form the foundation of a European medical tradition. Ayurveda has withstood the test of time, using all that nature provides not only to treat illness but to support healthy living as well. The word itself breaks down to mean "life" or "longevity" (ayur) and "knowledge" or "wisdom" (veda).

Ayurvedic theory is based on determining an individual's unique type or constitution and using foods, herbs, purgatives, rubbing oils and herbal pastes, massage, meditation, yoga, and lifestyle adjustments to construct a harmonious life. The practice of Ayurveda is becoming increasingly popular in the Western world. It offers a holistic approach, based on the understanding that no single agent by itself causes disease or brings health. Many new books on Ayurveda are available in English, and Ayurvedic treatment centers are opening throughout the United States and Europe.

For the past six years I have used Ayurvedic principles in my life, preparing meals and choosing particular spices and essential oils for their harmonizing qualities. I have found it to be an effective means of warding off or reducing the severity of colds and flus, as well as an excellent way to maintain my health and vitality. I have been fortunate to have my dear friend Candis Cantin Packard, an Ayurvedic practitioner, as a teacher. I have also learned from Ayurvedic students at the Maharishi University in Iowa, and their study of the qualities of various essential oils, and from Deepak Chopra's use of essential oils in his Ayurvedic treatment centers in San Diego and La Jolla, California.

The basic concepts of Ayurvedic theory make it a natural complement to aromatherapy. Ayurveda recognizes plants as "receptacles of light" and teaches that their "seven hundred natures" have the power to make whole that which has been hurt. An Ayurvedic physician concentrates on observation of the patient, and determining patterns of imbalance rather than diagnosis of a specific disease. By determining the constitution of the individual, he is able to deduce inherent strengths, weaknesses, and tendencies. The foundation of Ayurvedic theory lies in the manifestation of the three humors, referred to as "doshas." The doshas represent life force, and Ayurveda views each individual as a composite of the three doshas. The quality and relative balance of these forces within an individual determines health and disease. When these forces act harmoniously, we have health. When the doshas are in conflict or imbalance, we have illness. Specific symptoms indicate which of the doshas is deficient or excessive.

The unique combination of an individual's doshas comprise the "prikriti" or constitution. No two people will have the same prikriti. The following survey will help you determine your personal prikriti. You will no doubt find the influence of all three doshas, with one dominating your constitution. We are all combinations of the different doshas. For example, I am a kapha with a little bit of vata and a smaller amount of pitta. So I would be called a K-3, V-2, P-1. Some people are tridoshic, which means a balance of all three. That would abbreviate to V-2, P-2, K-2.

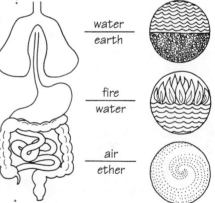

The Ayurvedic approach to health is based on a correspondence between body systems and constitutions with the basic elements of air, fire, water, earth, and ether.

THE THREE DOSHAS

Dosha	Elements	Quality	Constitution
Vata	Air & ether	Life	Cold, dry, and irregular
Pitta	Fire & water	Light	Hot, oily, and irritable
Kapha	Water & earth	Love	Cold, wet, and stable

VATA

The elements of vata are ether and air. The quality of vata is life. The vata body type is thin and wiry. You will rarely see an overweight vata; they are usually the people you see out jogging. They tend to have delicate, well-defined facial features and cool, dry skin. The vata constitution is both changeable and flexible, not only in body but also in mind. Vatas are unpredictable, often erratic, with a need to burn off nervous energy. They are also enthusiastic, impulsive, and moody. They conceptualize brilliantly but often have trouble following through. As with most everything in their lives, vatas' eating and sleeping habits are irregular, and they are prone to anxiety, worry, and insomnia. Vata in excess makes you ungrounded, spaced out, and unrealistic. The vata pulse is thin and fast and is said to "slither like a cobra." Vatas need moisture and lubrication. Vata headaches are relieved with warm sesame oil enemas. Dryness increases vata.

Vata Checklist

Score 1 point for each statement that applies to you most or some of the time.

- ❏ My bones tend to stick out with protruding points.
- ❏ My bones and joints make cracking noises.
- ❏ I tend to be underweight.
- ❏ My skin is usually very dry.
- ❏ I have cold hands and feet.
- ❏ I used to bite my nails.
- ❏ I have had chapped dry lips, eczema, or psoriasis.
- ❏ My hair feels coarse and gets split ends.
- ❏ My nails are dry and brittle or have ridges.
- ❏ I have sensitive teeth.

VATA OILS

Vata benefits from essential oils that have a warming and stimulating action, such as clove, cinnamon, cypress, galangal, melissa, wintergreen, and ud.

Vata may be irritated by fragrances that are too strong or perfumy. Fragrant oils that are grounding for vata include sandalwood, rose, jasmine, and spikenard.

Beneficial carrier oils for vata are sesame and hazelnut.

- ❏ My tongue has a very thin grayish coating.
- ❏ If I forget to eat I sometimes feel dizzy and weak.
- ❏ I like to eat sweets.
- ❏ I get constipated and full of gas sometimes.
- ❏ I enjoy activities like running or dancing.
- ❏ I tire out easily after exerting myself.
- ❏ I fantasize about sex.
- ❏ I sleep lightly and sometimes wake up or toss and turn in my sleep.
- ❏ I have nightmares or insomnia.
- ❏ I don't like cold, windy weather.
- ❏ My emotions are changeable.
- ❏ My mind is very fast, and so is my speech.
- ❏ Sometimes I have a hard time making a decision.
- ❏ I feel spacey sometimes.

Score for Vata _____

PITTA

The elements of pitta are fire and water. The quality of pitta is light. The pitta body type is a medium build, well proportioned and usually more muscular than the other types. Pittas' weight will often fluctuate, but they are more likely to gain weight. Pittas are quick, intelligent, and predictable. Efficient and businesslike, they tend to be highly organized and have regular eating and sleeping habits. They are passionate about things they care about, critical, often impatient, and easily angered. Pittas tends to heat up easily, sweat quickly, and become thirsty often. They suffer from rashes, fever, diarrhea, stomach ulcers, and hemorrhoids. Pitta in excess causes aggression and anger. It can cause one to become overly critical, blaming others. The pitta pulse is full, regular, and strong. It is said to "jump like a frog." Pitta headaches are relieved by drinking aloe vera gel. Anything hot increases pitta.

PITTA OILS

Pitta benefits from the cooling and calming effect of floral scents, such as champa, jasmine, rose, honeysuckle, violet, and mimosa.

Applied to the Third Eye, sandalwood is the best oil for pitta. Other cooling oils beneficial to pitta when applied to the head are lavender, mint, hina, and vetiver.

The first choice for a pitta carrier oil is olive or sunflower oil.

Pitta Checklist

Score 1 point for each statement that applies to you.

❏ My body is pretty well proportioned.
❏ I have a muscular, athletic build.
❏ My weight is usually average.
❏ My skin is warm and at times a bit ruddy.
❏ I sometimes find myself impatient or annoyed with other people.
❏ I get rashes or my skin breaks out.
❏ My hair is red or has a little red in it.
❏ I occasionally suffer from indigestion.
❏ My fingernails are strong, pinkish, and well shaped.
❏ My eyes sometimes become red and irritated.
❏ My tongue color is reddish with a yellow coating.
❏ I occasionally get canker sores or bleeding gums.
❏ My mouth sometimes tastes metallic or sour in the morning.
❏ I sometimes have a huge appetite.
❏ I am very well organized.
❏ I get uncomfortable if I skip a meal or if it is delayed.
❏ I love to eat ice cream.
❏ When I eat hot, spicy foods, I sweat.
❏ I drink a lot of liquids.
❏ I have regular bowel habits.
❏ I am extremely active; I enjoy lots of physical activities.
❏ I am very romantic and have a healthy sex drive.
❏ I sleep lightly, but if I wake up I can usually go back to sleep.
❏ If my desires are thwarted, my anger flares up.
Score for Pitta _____

KAPHA

The kapha elements are water and earth. The kapha quality is love. The kapha body type is solid and heavy. Kaphas are often overweight or on a diet. They love to eat, have slow digestion, and are reluctant to exercise. Kaphas love peace and comfort. They are relaxed and slow to anger. They are reluctant to face conflict, but are stubborn and will stand their ground if pushed. Kaphas are heavy sleepers and love to sleep in. They have oily skin and hair, and are prone to high cholesterol, congested lymph nodes, constipation, allergies, and gall-bladder and sinus problems. Kapha in excess causes dullness and lethargy. It can cause you to become passive, daydreamy, and overly dependent. A kapha pulse is slow and rhythmic; it is said to beat smoothly "like a swan." Kapha headaches can be remedied by inhalations of eucalyptus oil in hot steam. Anything heavy increases kapha.

Kapha Checklist

Score 1 point for each statement that applies to you.

❏ I have a large frame.
❏ I have a heavy bone structure.
❏ I tend to gain weight easily.
❏ It is very difficult for me to lose weight, except if I fast.
❏ My skin is very soft and usually very clear and smooth.
❏ My hair is very thick and sometimes oily.
❏ I have strong, large fingernails.
❏ People always notice my large, soft eyes.
❏ My teeth are very even.
❏ My tongue sometimes has a thick whitish coating.
❏ I fall asleep easily and usually sleep well.
❏ I sometimes crave sweet or fatty foods.

KAPHA OILS

Kapha does best with essential oils that are warm, mildly stimulating, and expectorant, such as rosemary, sage, spruce, pine, myrrh, basil, camphor, patchouli, cinnamon, ginger, black pepper, kewda, mitti, and trifolia.

The best carrier oils for kapha are almond, apricot, and flaxseed.

- ❏ I can skip meals without a problem.
- ❏ I am lazy and have to push myself to do any activities.
- ❏ If I am in good shape, I have a lot of endurance.
- ❏ I have a hard time waking up in the morning.
- ❏ I sometimes experience bloating and water retention.
- ❏ I am very loving and have a steady sex drive.
- ❏ I tend to be very easygoing by nature.
- ❏ Once aroused I can become very intense.
- ❏ I dislike arguments and confrontations.
- ❏ I am slow to express my ideas.
- ❏ I seldom get angry.
- ❏ I get attached and greedy sometimes.

Score for Kapha _____

AYURVEDIC ANOINTING

Ayurvedic theory prescribes daily massage or self-massage of the body with oils to balance the doshas. Ayurvedic theory can guide the aromatherapist in selecting the right oils to fit the particular person and special needs. Once you decide which dosha you wish to affect, you can choose the appropriate oils and use them in traditional aromatherapy applications or use them to enhance Ayurvedic therapies.

Shiro dhara is a unique Ayurvedic treatment that consists of pouring a fine, continuous stream of warm sesame oil over the forehead. The addition of highly active essential oils to a shiro dhara treatment will enhance its positive results and provide additional benefits.

The bridge of loose skin between your toes is full of reflex areas, as are the insides of the nostrils and the ears. Massaging these areas with a few drops of essential oil diluted in a small amount of carrier oil is very calming and balancing to the prikriti. Essential oils can also be placed over the chakras to balance the doshas and clear the auric field.

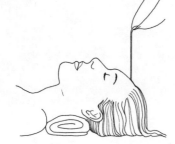

The Ayurvedic practice of shiro dhara seeks to balance the three doshas by pouring a fine stream of warmed sesame oil over the forehead to stimulate the Third Eye.

Ayurvedic Anointing Blends

These formulas are designed to balance the doshas. Once you've determined the dosha you wish to enhance, combine all ingredients in a 30 or 60 ml (1 or 2 ounce) bottle, and shake well. Apply as a massage oil.

Vata Blend

- 10 drops sandalwood essential oil
- 2 drops cinnamon essential oil
- 4 drops rose essential oil
- 30 ml (1 ounce) hazelnut oil
- 30 ml (1 ounce) sesame oil

Vata-Kapha Blend

- 10 drops sandalwood essential oil
- 5 drops spruce essential oil
- 10 drops cypress essential oil
- 30 ml (1 ounce) sesame oil
- 30 ml (1 ounce) almond oil

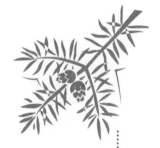

Vata-Pitta Blend

- 10 drops sandalwood essential oil
- 6 drops patchouli essential oil
- 12 drops cedarwood essential oil
- 30 ml (1 ounce) sesame oil
- 30 ml (1 ounce) almond oil

Pitta Blend

- 10 drops sandalwood essential oil
- 8 drops lavender essential oil
- 2 drops rose essential oil
- 2 drops violet leaf essential oil
- 30 ml (1 ounce) olive oil

Pitta-Vata Blend

20 drops orange essential oil
 4 drops cinnamon essential oil
 5 drops cardamon essential oil
 4 drops jasmine essential oil
30 ml (1 ounce) sesame oil
30 ml (1 ounce) sunflower oil

Pitta-Kapha Blend

20 drops orange essential oil
 8 drops bergamot essential oil
 2 drops ylang ylang essential oil
25 ml (5 tablespoons) coconut oil
 5 ml (1 teaspoon) flaxseed oil

Kapha Blend

20 drops rosemary essential oil
10 drops spruce essential oil
10 drops basil essential oil
30 ml (1 ounce) almond oil

Kapha-Pitta Blend

10 drops orange essential oil
 5 drops myrrh essential oil
 5 drops vetiver essential oil
 5 drops patchouli essential oil
30 ml (1 ounce) apricot oil
30 ml (1 ounce) almond oil

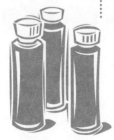

YOGA AND AROMATHERAPY

The discipline of yoga is closely allied with Ayurveda. Yoga, which means "union," is more than just a series of body postures that increase flexibility. The path of yoga calls for an intense awareness of mind and body so that our actions arise from a balanced and pure motive.

I have noticed that people in the Western world tend to ignore or misinterpret subtle information from their physical bodies. Aches and pains, stiffness and weakness, are often ignored until they manifest into a disease. Then the person turns to a doctor and demands a fast cure. When we really listen to our bodies, as yoga practice will encourage, we will recognize when something is not right, and often we will intuitively seek appropriate curative therapies.

The burning of sandalwood incense has traditionally been a part of yoga practice. When you arrive at a temple, asana hall, or ashram you will usually smell sandalwood, champa, or some other type of incense burning. The particular brand and type of incense can be very important in creating a scent memory for yoga students. They will always associate that particular scent with their yoga instructor and with the spiritual and physical growth they experience with their yoga practice.

It is not uncommon for people who practice yoga to create a ritual around it. They may practice always in the same place in the house, using a special rug or mat that is reserved strictly for yoga. There is often a photo of a yoga instructor or guru on the wall, along with an incense burner or aromatherapy diffuser.

These rituals enhance the practice of yoga by isolating the experience and making it important to the subconscious as well as the conscious mind. Incorporating a scent memory into any ritual defines it as important and worthy of spiritual focus. A wonderful aromatic ritual to combine with your yoga practice is to begin your session by anointing your forehead with sandalwood or a paste of sandalwood and amber.

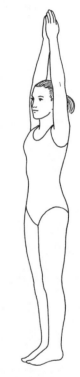

Aromatherapy can be used to help the mind focus and the body relax during yoga practice.

The following blends are excellent to diffuse in the early morning before a yoga class.

Formula 1

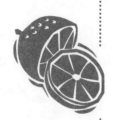

    12 *drops orange essential oil*
     4 *drops clove essential oil*
     4 *drops ylang ylang essential oil*

Formula 2

    10 *drops orange essential oil*
     4 *drops bergamot essential oil*
     4 *drops lemon essential oil*
     4 *drops lime essential oil*

THE FOUR HUMORS AND CORRESPONDING OILS

The idea of assessing health concerns and developing remedies based on body type and personality is not unique to the East. In Western medicine, the Greek physician Hippocrates developed the concept of the four humors in the fourth century B.C. The theory was that all disease could be understood as a problem with the "humors," or an imbalance related to the natural tendency of a particular humor, or body and personality type. The chart on the facing page illustrates how these four humors were illustrated and described.

I see remarkable similarities in this analysis to the Ayurvedic "temperaments," as well as to the four elements — fire, water, earth, and air — that are the base for ancient alchemy, astrology, and Chinese medicine. I have taken the liberty of combining the four humors, Ayurvedic concepts, and astrological elements in this chart.

THE FOUR HUMORS
(with Ayurvedic Types)

**LYMPHATIC/
PHLEGMATIC**

KAPHA (water + earth)

(negative)

**NERVOUS/
MELANCHOLIC**

Appearance: Square, large face. Chin wider than forehead. Hands are long, feel soft and damp, with cold palms. Body larger below the waist. Lips well marked.

Temperament: Steady, slow, and gentle people who talk softly and have large eyes. When depressed, these personalities tend to get stuck and congested, constipated, and can get abscesses. Like to eat sweets and fats.

Element: Earth

Astrological signs: Taurus, Capricorn, Virgo

Appearance: Heart- or triangle-shaped face with small chin. Cold hands, thin, pointed fingers, graceful movements of the hands. Quick eyes.

Temperament: Rapid speech. Happiest when they're in love. When not in love, become emotionally depressed and chest closes up. Tend to suppress emotions and hold on to hurt. Don't eat breakfast, drink a lot of coffee, may grind teeth. Tire quickly.

Element: Water

Astrological signs: Scorpio, Cancer, Pisces

neutral/
balance

Appearance: Squarish face with round nose. Hands are thick and feel hot and humid. Big chest.

Temperament: These people are always hot and perspire easily. Face is red. Quick to anger and tend to yell a lot. Don't hold grudges. Tend to be excessive in eating and drinking. Suffer from mental anxiety.

Element: Air

Astrological signs: Libra, Gemini, Aquarius

Appearance: Well-proportioned, rectangular face. Hands feel hot and dry. Skin tends to be yellow.

Temperament: Active, type "A" personality. Very busy and sporty. Executive types, always traveling. Eat fast. Tend to get fevers, rashes, and infection when run down.

Element: Fire

Astrological signs: Sagittarius, Aries, Leo

**SANGUINE/
MENTAL**

**VATA
(air + ether)**

(positive)

**PITTA
(fire + water)**

**CHOLERIC/
BILIOUS**

Using the Hippocratic Four Humors Chart as a backdrop, Pierre Franchomme, a French essential oil researcher, created a modern version of this chart, mapping out the essential oil groups that correspond to each humor or personality type. The essential oils are grouped by their main chemical constituents (as described in Chapter 3).

LYMPHATIC/
PHLEGMATIC

KAPHA (water + earth)

↑

(negative)

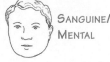

NERVOUS/
MELANCHOLIC

ALDEHYDES — soothing on the nervous system. Good for insomnia, stress, skin irritants. Antiseptic, antiviral, fungicidal, insecticidal.
Essential oils: lemongrass, lemon verbena, *Eucalyptus citriodora*
Associated colors: yellow and light green

ESTERS — the most user-friendly oils. Balancing, calming, and energizing. Good for skin care. Antiseptic.
Essential oils: lavender, clary sage, bergamot, geranium, Roman chamomile
Associated color: lavender

SESQUITERPENES — most soothing and sedating. Antiallergenic, antiseptic, antirheumatic. Good for burns and severe skin surface damage.
Essential oils: German chamomile, yarrow, celery seed, artemisia
Associated colors: light blue to indigo

KETONES — most aggressive and potentially toxic. Antitumor, detoxifying. In large amounts, toxic to liver and nervous system. Antiseptic, bactericidal, antiviral.
Essential Oils: sage, pennyroyal, rosemary, wormwood, hyssop
Associated color: green

neutral/ balance

ALCOHOLS — largest and most popular group. Antiseptic, astringent, fungicidal, sedative. Aphrodisiacs.
Essential oils: clary sage, sandalwood, MQV, myrtle, *Eucalyptus radiata*, tea tree, bois de rose, *Eucalyptus globulus*, peppermint, spearmint
Associated colors: turquoise, green, aqua

OXIDES — respiratory, expectorant, antiseptic, fungicidal.
Essential oils: niaouli, cajeput, myrtle, ravensara
Associated colors: green and blue

ETHERS — digestive, antiseptic, aperitif, antispasmodic. Licorice-tasting.
Essential oils: anise, fennel seed, tarragon, basil
Associated color: light green

PHENOLS — energizing and irritating to skin. Antiseptic, bactericidal, antimicrobial, antioxidant.
Essential oils: savory, oregano, thyme, clove, cinnamon
Associated colors: orange, red

TERPENES — most aggressive and stimulating. Bactericidal, antiseptic. Drying, astringent. Tonic, diuretic.
Essential oils: lemon, grapefruit, mandarin, lime, pine, juniper, black pepper, frankincense
Associated color: red

SANGUINE/
MENTAL

**VATA
(air + ether)**

(positive)

**PITTA
(fire + water)**

CHOLERIC/
BILIOUS

↓

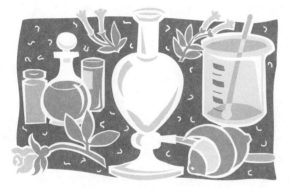

Mythology and
Aromatherapy

CHAPTER

In 1982, on the island of Crete in Greece, I was inspired to create some blends incorporating goddess mythology with aromatherapy. I have always been fascinated with the goddesses of Greek mythology. In ancient myths, the stories of the goddesses are invariably interwoven with the history of the flowers and plants of the earth. I felt that by using aromatherapy blends inspired by the female archetypes represented in goddess mythology, women could embody the energy of the myth in their own lives. The fusion of goddess mythology and aromatherapy is represented in the following blends, each dedicated to a different goddess.

ATHENA

Athens was named for this goddess born of Zeus. She had no mother, but leaped full grown from the head of her father. Fierce and ruthless, Athena was her father's favorite daughter (he had three) and was considered a protector of civilization. According to legend, Athena won her city with the gift of an olive tree, which became the most prized tree in all of Greece. Athena's gift became a symbol of peace for time immemorial and has since been treasured for both its food and the healing properties of its oil and leaves.

Today Athena exemplifies the career woman — the successful, intellectual woman who can hold her own working with men. Using her mind exhaustively, she sometimes loses touch with her own sensuality. The Athena blend helps this type of woman reintegrate her physical, mental, and spiritual bodies. It helps her to achieve wholeness and tap into a fuller power.

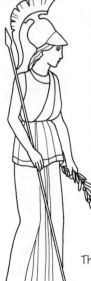

The goddess Athena represents the highly intellectual woman.

Athena Blend Body Oil

60 ml (2 ounces) grapeseed oil
30 ml (1 ounce) apricot oil
30 ml (1 ounce) macadamia, avocado, or rose hip oil
  Lavender essential oil
  Geranium essential oil
  Sweet marjoram essential oil
  Clary sage essential oil
  Blue chamomile essential oil

Mix the carrier oils in a 120 ml (4 ounce) dark glass bottle and add a total of 20 to 30 drops of a combination of the essential oils.
To use: After a shower or bath, lightly towel-dry and, while your pores are still open, apply the oil. Start at the feet and work up. The oil will mix with the water left on the surface of your skin to form a creamy lotion.

Athena's Milk and Honey Bath

100 g (3½ ounces) sea salt
100 g (3½ ounces) Epsom salts
  1 liter (quart) milk
450 g (1 pound) honey

1. Combine sea salt and Epsom salts in a jar and mix well. Pour the salts into the bathtub and run hot water over them to dissolve.
2. While the bath continues filling, heat the milk in a saucepan (taking care not to boil it), then mix the honey into the hot milk.
3. Pour the milk-and-honey mixture into the bath just before entering and relax for at least 20 minutes, adding hot water as needed to keep the temperature comfortable. You will emerge from this bath with the silken skin of a goddess.

BENEFITS OF ATHENA BLEND

To combat negative thoughts that deplete feminine energy or to relieve conflicting and obsessive thoughts related to career and work, use an Athena blend as a massage or body oil.

APHRODITE

Aphrodite is the goddess of love and beauty. According to myth, she sprang from the foam of the sea, fully formed, upon a giant shell. Unlike other goddesses, Aphrodite was free to choose her lover. She gave birth to Eros, god of love. The Aphrodite archetype governs a woman's enjoyment of love, beauty, sexuality, and sensuality. Creative work is also fueled by the intense passions of Aphrodite. Some women feel her influence most at the time of ovulation, when the act of love is most likely to result in pregnancy. It is from her name that we get the word *aphrodisiac*. An Aphrodite blend is made up of oils that have aphrodisiac properties.

APHRODITE BLEND BODY OIL

60 ml (2 ounces) grapeseed oil
30 ml (1 ounce) apricot oil
30 ml (1 ounce) macadamia, avocado, or rose hip oil
  Ylang ylang essential oil
  Orange essential oil
  Vanilla essential oil
  Jasmine essential oil
  Sandalwood essential oil
  Neroli essential oil

Mix the carrier oils in a 120 ml (4 ounce) dark glass bottle and add a total of 20 to 30 drops of a combination of the essential oils.
To use: To promote creativity or to relieve stress and nurture your sensual, sexual nature, use an Aphrodite blend as a massage or body oil. After a shower or bath, lightly towel-dry and, while your pores are still open, apply the oil. Start at the feet and work up. The oil will mix with the water left on the surface of your skin to form a creamy lotion.

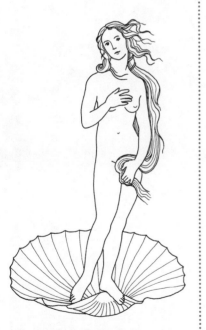

The goddess Aphrodite is synonymous with love and beauty.

APHRODITE'S MILK AND FLOWER BATH

- 1 liter (quart) milk
- 10 drops orange essential oil
- 6 drops ylang ylang essential oil
- 2 drops jasmine essential oil
- 4 drops neroli essential oil
- 4 drops sandalwood essential oil

While the bath is filling, heat the milk in a saucepan (taking care not to boil it) and mix the essential oils into the warm milk.
To use: Pour the milk-and-oil mixture into the bath just before entering and relax for at least 20 minutes, adding hot water as needed to keep the temperature comfortable. Light a few candles, and add a vase of fresh flowers to make this a very special bath.

ATLANTIA

Atlantia is the athletic woman, one of the Amazons. Her father, disappointed that the infant Atlantia was not a boy, left her in the wild to die of cold and hunger. But Atlantia was adopted by a she-bear and grew to be an active and daring little girl. Her athletic prowess attracted many suitors, and Atlantia, confident that no man could equal her fleetness of foot, agreed to marry any man who could beat her in a footrace. Hippomenes loved Atlantia and sought the assistance of Aphrodite in winning her. Aphrodite, in the interest of true love, provided Hippomenes with three golden apples with which to distract Atlantia during the race, so that he could win her hand through trickery. In other legends, Atlantia was a warrior priestess. Her archetype rules over aerobic activity and physical endurance. Women under the guidance of Atlantia excel in sports.

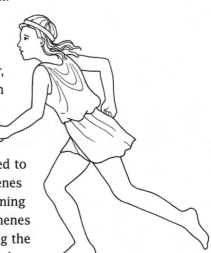

The goddess Atlantia is associated with qualities of physical endurance and an enjoyment of sports.

ATLANTIA BLEND OIL

60 ml (2 ounces) grapeseed oil
30 ml (1 ounce) apricot oil
30 ml (1 ounce) macadamia, avocado, or rose hip oil
  Orange essential oil
  Grapefruit essential oil
  Lemon essential oil
  Lemongrass essential oil
  Lime essential oil

Mix the carrier oils in a 120 ml (4 ounce) dark glass bottle and add a total of 20 to 30 drops of a combination of the essential oils.
To use: To promote aerobic activity, use an Atlantia blend as a massage or body oil. After a shower or bath, lightly towel-dry and, while your pores are still open, apply the oil. Start at the feet and work up. The oil will mix with the water left on the surface of your skin to form a creamy lotion. Or add 10 to 15 drops of an Atlantia blend to a hot bath for an invigorating soak.

ARTEMIS

Artemis was a goddess of the hunt, a lover of the woods and the wild chase over the mountains. Twin sister to Apollo, she was a child of nature, a protectress of dewy youth. An emotional distance is characteristic of the archetypal Artemis woman. She is often so focused on her own aims that she fails to notice the feelings of those around her. Artemis needs to hear and heed others. Named for this goddess, the *Artemisia arborescens* plant is a remarkable healer. Even the most impossible rashes seem to respond to frequent applications and misting with floral waters of artemis. This special blend of aromatics is for delicate skin that has been overexposed to the sun and damaged by the elements.

Artemis, the goddess of the hunt, represents a focused, goal-oriented woman, who may be out of touch with her emotions.

ARTEMISIA BLEND OIL

60 ml (2 ounces) grapeseed oil

30 ml (1 ounce) apricot oil

30 ml (1 ounce) macadamia, avocado, or rose hip oil

   Artemisia douglasiana or *A. californica* essential oil

   A. arborescens essential oil

   Rose essential oil

   Lavender essential oil

Mix the carrier oils in a 120 ml (4 ounce) dark glass bottle and add a total of 20 to 30 drops of a combination of the essential oils.
To use: To heal and protect damaged skin, use an Artemisia blend as a facial or body oil. Add 10 to 15 drops of an Artemisia blend to a hot bath to soothe irritated skin and promote a dewy, youthful glow. After a shower or bath, lightly towel-dry and, while your pores are still open, place 3 to 5 drops on your stomach and massage lightly, moving up and over the breast and neck area. As the oil mixes with the moisture on the surface of your skin to form a creamy lotion, extend your strokes to bring the lotion onto your face. This will leave you with a nice protective shield, like a soft second skin.

PSYCHE

Psyche was the most beautiful of three sisters. To prevent a prophecy of her father's destruction from fulfilling itself, Psyche was taken to a high mountain and thrown to her death. But an enormous winged creature swooped her up and took her to his castle. Psyche awoke to find herself in a wonderful palace, visited by a mysterious lover. Eros, the god of love, kept his identity a secret by visiting Psyche only under cover of darkness. When Psyche pined for her two sisters, Eros agreed to let them visit. The sisters were

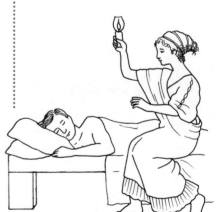

The goddess Psyche represents the pain and beauty of erotic love.

jealous of Psyche and convinced her that her lover must be an ugly old man. At the urging of the jealous sisters, Psyche lit an oil lamp to reveal Eros in his sleep. Overcome at his handsomeness, she dropped the lamp, burning his chest with the hot oil. In anger he swore she would never again gaze upon him and flew away. Poor wretched Psyche, now pregnant, wandered the earth in search of her beloved Eros. All of nature wanted to help to reunite these two, for Psyche held inside her the "love child" of her match with Eros. The lovers were eventually reunited, following the twin birth of the Unicorn and Pegasus, the offspring of this fabled pair. Psyche represents the innocence, pain, and beauty of erotic love. Eros is an anagram of *rose.*

PSYCHE BLEND OIL

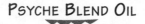

60 ml (2 ounces) grapeseed oil
30 ml (1 ounce) apricot oil
30 ml (1 ounce) macadamia, avocado, or rose hip oil
   Bois de rose essential oil
   Orange essential oil
   Patchouli essential oil
   Rose essential oil
   Cinnamon essential oil
   Tonka essential oil

Mix the carrier oils in a 120 ml (4 ounce) dark glass bottle and add a total of 20 to 30 drops of a combination of the essential oils.
To use: Use this very sensuous blend as a massage or body oil. After a shower or bath, lightly towel-dry and, while your pores are still open, apply the oil. Start at the feet and work up. The oil will mix with the water left on the surface of your skin to form a creamy lotion.

PSYCHE'S HOT OIL BATH

10 drops orange essential oil
6 drops bois de rose essential oil
4 drops patchouli essential oil
2 drops cinnamon essential oil
2 drops rose essential oil

6 drops cedarwood
   essential oil
20 ml (4 teaspoons)
   apricot oil

While the bath is filling, pour the apricot oil into a cup (235 ml) of hot water and add the essential oils.

To use: Pour the oil mixture into the bath just before entering and relax for at least 20 minutes, adding hot water as needed. Light a candle to help soothe the pain of a lonely heart.

DEMETER BLEND

Demeter was the goddess of the hearth. A wife and mother, Demeter is the archetype of the maternal woman. She is also considered the Crone, a wise woman honored for her experience and knowledge.

60 ml (2 ounces) grapeseed oil
30 ml (1 ounce) apricot oil
30 ml (1 ounce) macadamia,
   avocado, or rose hip oil

Cypress essential oil
Juniper essential oil
Lemon essential oil
Black pepper essential oil

Mix the carrier oils in a 120 ml (4 ounce) dark glass bottle and add a total of 20 to 30 drops of a combination of the essential oils.

To use: Use as a massage or body oil to combat cellulite and weight gain caused by lack of exercise. After a shower or bath, lightly towel-dry and, while your pores are still open, apply the oil. Start at the feet and work up. The oil will mix with the water left on the surface of your skin to form a creamy lotion. Or add 10 to 15 drops of a Demeter blend to a hot bath to promote healthy circulation.

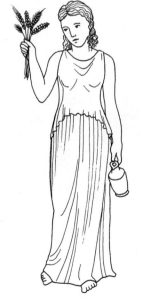

Demeter is noted for her maternal instincts and wisdom.

CELTIC GODDESS BLEND

60 ml (2 ounces) grapeseed oil
30 ml (1 ounce) apricot oil
30 ml (1 ounce) macadamia,
    avocado, or rose hip oil

Patchouli essential oil
Lemon essential oil
Lemongrass essential oil
Ylang ylang essential oil

Mix the carrier oils in a 120 ml (4 ounce) dark glass bottle and add a total of 20 to 30 drops of a combination of the essential oils.

To use: Use as a massage or body oil, or add 10 to 15 drops to a tub of hot water for a bath fit for a Celtic goddess.

ANOINTING WITH OILS

The ritual of anointing with oils has held a tremendous amount of symbolism throughout history. The ritual carries the concept of benediction, of bestowing divine blessing and giving grace to the soul. In ancient Egyptian temples, high priestesses performed ritual anointings as they passed on their wisdom in sacred ceremonies. Ritual anointing is employed in the coronation of kings, in the crowning of bishops, cardinals, and popes, and in the appointment of other revered spiritual leaders.

Anointing can be very spiritually energizing. When you anoint with oils, you are giving a blessing. Your state of mind and your sincerity are of great importance. Anointment rituals are shared for purely spiritual reasons, as healing ceremonies, or to achieve a specific physical or psychological state.

Using Essential Oils

You can create your own anointing rituals to visualize and manifest change and growth in your life. Whether your ritual is as simple as a dab of oil on your forehead combined with an affirmation, or an

Using Essential Oils for Anointing

Oil	Purpose/Effect	Body Part to Apply On
Amber	Romantic love, illusions about love	Inner wrists
Artemisia	Connect to nature spirits, animal totem spirits, stimulate dream journey	Inhale
Frankincense	Spiritual truth, protection from negative influences, meditation to invoke the solar goddess, clairvoyance	Inhale or crown of head
Geranium	Activate and balance the body and emotions	Back
Jasmine	Aphrodisiac, mood elevating, happiness	Head and neck area
Lavender	Soothe, cleanse, and calm the psyche	Anywhere on the body; in the bath
Myrrh	Magical, psychic healing, uplifting, purifying	Inhale or crown of head
Neroli	Sleep inducing, trance inducing, enhances dream states	Abdomen, hara, second chakra area
Oakmoss	Prosperity rituals	Palms of the hands
Patchouli	Grounding, processing past experiences, clear visions	Sacrum
Rose	Loving, soothing, harmonious relationships	Over heart area
Sandalwood	Sensual and grounding, meditation, soothe the mind	Temples, Third Eye
Spikenard	Invokes ancient visions, prepares the psyche for shocks, coping with emotional or physical traumas	All chakra points
St.-John's-wort	Balances emotional wounds	Crown of head
Ud	To reach higher spiritual states of being, connect with the spirit world	Inner earlobe

elaborate ceremony with many props, prayers, and players, the above chart will help you select the appropriate oils for your anointing. These recommendations are taken from the ancient tradition of anointing as part of a spiritual discipline. To prepare anointing oils, start with a 1-ounce (30 ml) bottle of jojoba oil and add up to 20 drops of essential oil. Shake the bottle and focus upon your intentions for this oil and the purpose of the anointing.

SUFI HEALING

Sufis (followers of a form of Islamic mysticism) believe that all illness has a spiritual cause, so they use aromatic oils for spiritual healing. Following are a few very special Sufi blends designed to address various emotional issues when applied to one of the seven chakras, or energy centers, of the body. Any of these blends can be mixed into ½ tablespoon (7½ ml) of jojoba oil and stored in a dark bottle.

CHAKRA BLENDS

Base Chakra Blend

    2 drops jasmine essential oil
    2 drops rose essential oil
    5 drops frankincense essential oil

Use: For emotional insecurity, selfish behavior, aggression, sexual perversion, depression, and fear.

Second Chakra Blend

    1 gram amber essential oil
   10 drops sandalwood essential oil
    4 drops hina essential oil

Use: For all emotional trauma, lack of concentration and energy.

Third Chakra Blend

    4 drops rose essential oil
   10 drops frankincense essential oil
    2 drops violet essential oil

Use: For selfishness, self-doubt, depression, weeping, and suicidal thoughts.

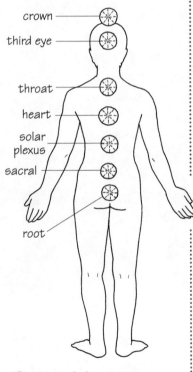

crown

third eye

throat

heart

solar plexus

sacral

root

The seven chakras, or energy centers, of the body are focal points for anointing the body with oils in the Sufi tradition.

Fourth Chakra Blend

  4 drops jasmine essential oil
  6 drops sandalwood essential oil
  6 drops frankincense essential oil
  2 drops violet essential oil

Use: For excessive emotion, fear of failure, financial instability, self-doubt, and extreme anger.

Fifth Chakra Blend

  3 drops rose essential oil
  6 drops sandalwood essential oil
  2 drops violet essential oil

Use: For selfishness, arrogance, degrading others, and forgetfulness.

Sixth Chakra Blend

  10 drops sandalwood essential oil
  2 drops ud essential oil
  4 drops hina essential oil

Use: For oversensitivity, forgetfulness, disconnection with reality, lack of life force.

Seventh Chakra Blend

  5 drops rose essential oil
20–25 drops rose amber essential oil

Use: For states of ecstasy, silence, or incoherence.

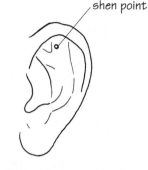

shen point

The shen point, located in the upper fold of the ear, is a major brain point in acupuncture and ear acupressure. The Sufis believe it to be a place that stimulates divine connection and serves as a gateway to the gods, and anoint it with a few drops of oil.

AROMATHERAPY AND THE ZODIAC

According to astrological theory, plants take on the characteristics of the planets that rule them. For example, the sun is the ruler of orange fruits and blossoms, and of plants that grow in the hot desert, such as frankincense and myrrh. Plants also take on the symbology of the different parts of the body that they are meant to heal.

To create your own personal astrological blend, choose oils from the signs that dominate your chart. Then try mixing just a few drops of each oil into a base of jojoba oil. For example, if you are a Taurus with Libra rising and a Gemini moon, you could mix 2 drops of ylang ylang, 2 drops of rose, 2 drops of geranium, 2 drops of palmarosa, and 4 drops of lavender.

ESSENTIAL OIL BLENDS FOR ASTROLOGICAL SIGNS

Sign	Element	Essential Oils
Aries	Fire	Black pepper, basil, ginger, coriander, mugwort
Taurus	Earth	Ylang ylang, rose, honeysuckle, thyme, mints
Gemini	Air	Caraway, carrot, fennel, lavender, marjoram
Cancer	Water	Chamomile, artemesia, yarrow, violet, clary sage
Leo	Fire	Frankincense, myrrh, angelica, orange, neroli
Virgo	Earth	Rosemary, lavender, cypress, melissa, peppermint
Libra	Air	Geranium, palmarosa, rose, pine, eucalyptus
Scorpio	Water	Black pepper, mugwort, cardamom, pennyroyal
Sagittarius	Fire	Melissa, cedar, nutmeg, birch, hyssop, clove
Capricorn	Earth	Jasmine, vetiver, oakmoss, wintergreen, patchouli
Aquarius	Air	Cypress, mimosa, sassafras, vanilla
Pisces	Water	Sandalwood, clove, cinnamon, linden blossom

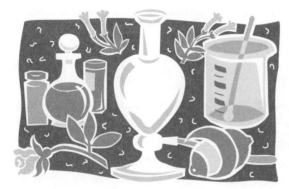

Aromatherapy
for Children
and Teenagers

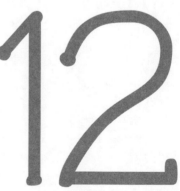

 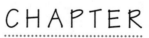

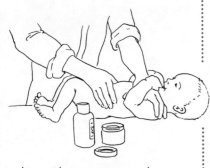

Aromatherapy massage is a wonderful way to give your baby the tactile stimulation and love he needs.

Those years when you are caring for newborns, toddlers, and children can be a very rewarding time to use aromatherapy. The childhood years are full of minor and major crises, and many times aromatherapy can help. You must always remember to dilute oils appropriately before administering them to children: Children are much more sensitive to essential oils than adults. Taking this extra sensitivity into consideration, along with a child's smaller size, usually means an appropriate child's dose would be one-quarter of an adult dose.

Baby Massage

Massaging your baby can be a most delightful experience for both of you. Touch is very important for small babies. Next to breast-feeding, massage is the most intimate contact you can have with your baby. It functions as a sensual bonding experience. Babies and children are extremely tactile, and frequent physical contact is crucially important for their survival. Hopefully your baby will get touched and massaged a lot.

SWEET BREATH BABY OIL

Here is an excellent choice for your baby's first massage oil.

> 10 drops lavender essential oil
> 4 drops neroli essential oil
> 2 drops Roman chamomile essential oil
> 120 ml (4 ounces) almond or apricot oil

Mix in a 120 ml (4 ounce) dark glass bottle and shake well.
To use: Warm the oil in your hands and lightly massage your baby all over with this oil following a bath. You will both benefit.

Calendula Infusion for Baby

Calendula has long been recognized for its soothing and healing properties. It was used extensively as a medicine during World War I when an American nurse, Gertrude Jekyll, instigated a campaign to grow and gather calendula to be used for dressing wounds. The plants were shipped to first-aid stations in France. Today the petals are a popular ingredient in ointments.

You can make a fine massage oil for your baby by infusing fresh calendula blossoms in oil. Pick fresh organically grown calendula flowers. Remove the stems and any bugs and blot the petals dry on paper towels before packing the flowers into a clean quart (l) jar that has been sterilized and completely dried. Cover the blossoms with almond or apricot oil and place a few layers of cheesecloth over the mouth of the jar, securing it with a rubber band. Leave the jar in a warm spot for two weeks, then strain the oil though the cheesecloth.

This infused oil also makes an excellent dressing for scraped knees, cut fingers, and insect bites.

BATH OIL FOR BABY

This bath oil blend is also very soothing for older children and effective for treating childhood insomnia.

    5 drops lavender essential oil
    2 drops chamomile essential oil
    30 ml (1 ounce) milk

Mix the lavender and chamomile into the milk.
To use: Stir into baby's bathwater for a mild, soothing bath.

TIPS ON SELECTING OILS

◆ Don't confuse calendula flowers — sometimes called pot marigolds — with the common garden variety of marigolds.

◆ Use Roman, German, or Moroccan blue chamomile, or Tanacetum annuum. These oils are very gentle. Avoid oils that are labeled "Wild Chamomile" or "Chamaemelum mixta." They are similar smelling but have a stimulating effect rather than the calming action the other chamomiles are noted for.

Safe Baby Powder

Baby powder is a classic baby product. It is soft and fragrant, soothing, and drying for little bottoms that have been overexposed to wet diapers. But the talc used in commercial baby powders can be harmful to your baby's tender lungs. Because it is virtually impossible to powder a baby's little body without dispersing minute particles into the air, I recommend eliminating all talcum-based products from the nursery. An effective, safe, and superior baby powder is simple to make.

BABY POWDER BLEND

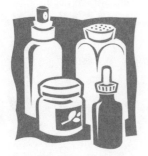

10 drops lavender essential oil
2 drops chamomile essential oil
60 g (2 ounces) white clay or cornstarch

Stir the oils into the clay or cornstarch.
To use: Keep in a powder shaker to use with diaper changes.

A Simple Colic Remedy

A colicky baby is an unhappy baby. Some babies never suffer from colic; others have only an occasional tummy ache. Count yourself lucky if you're the parent of one of these babies. But many healthy babies go through a colicky period during the first three months of life, when nothing seems to agree with them. Their little digestive systems seem unable to cope with all the new activity and they build up painful gas. Few things can make a new parent feel more helpless than trying to comfort a colicky baby who is crying in pain and rage.

Fennel is a colicky baby's best friend. Dilute 3 drops of fennel oil in a quart (l) of distilled water. One or 2 drops of this fennel water placed on the baby's tongue with an eyedropper should provide soothing relief for most colic and stomach upsets. You can substitute peppermint or dill for the fennel with similar effect.

Immunization Reactions

We immunize our children to protect them from the possibly devastating effects of some common childhood diseases. But occasionally children suffer a negative reaction from the very immunizations we hope will protect them. Usually these reactions are localized, with redness and swelling at the injection site, or generalized, with slight fever and viral symptoms. Although the reaction is probably not life threatening, it can make a baby very uncomfortable for a day or two.

IMMUNIZATION SOOTHER

5 drops geranium essential oil
5 drops sandalwood essential oil
30 ml (1 ounce) carrier oil

Combine all oils in a dark glass container.
Use: To relieve discomfort following immunizations, massage a small amount of this oil directly onto the injection site.

FORMULAS FOR TODDLERS

Toddlers are busy little folks with very active and curious minds. Most toddlers can run circles around their mothers and often seem to require less sleep than their exhausted parents crave. But in reality toddlers still need a good bit of quiet time. Sometimes they can use some help calming down.

Toddler's Massage Oil

    10 drops lavender essential oil
     4 drops marjoram essential oil
     2 drops ylang ylang essential oil
    60 ml (2 ounces) almond or apricot oil

Mix and store in a small, dark glass bottle.
To use: A gentle rub with this calming massage oil can help your toddler calm down and focus on some quiet activity.

Child's Body Powder

A light dusting with this body powder after the bath is a pleasure for any child, and the clay or cornstarch is so much safer for tender young lungs than the harsh talcs found in commercial products.

    10 drops lavender essential oil
     5 drops bergamot essential oil
     2 drops ylang ylang essential oil
    60 g (2 ounces) white clay or cornstarch

Stir the oils into the clay or cornstarch.
To use: Store in a widemouthed jar with a big fluffy puff for dusting on after the bath.

AROMATHERAPY FOR COMMON CHILDHOOD AILMENTS

The massive amount of antibiotics given to children in the United States since the 1950s is great disservice of modern allopathic medicine. The quick administration of antibiotics to treat minor illnesses actually undermines the body's natural ability to heal itself.

However, there are times when your child is ill and feeling miserable, and you feel desperate to provide some sort of relief.

Some essential oils are an effective alternative to antibiotic therapy, and many others actually complement and support the action of antibiotics. In France aromatherapy is taken far more seriously by mainstream medicine than anywhere else in the world. French pharmaceutical testing has demonstrated, for instance, that niaouli — marketed in France as a pharmaceutically pure essence called Gomenol — actually increases the activity of streptomycin and penicillin. French research also indicates that other essential oils high in terpineol, such as terebinth, pine, nutmeg, and marjoram, as well as turpentine derivatives, work well in conjunction with antibiotics.

EAR INFECTION FORMULA

Young children probably take more antibiotics to treat inner ear infections than for any other reason. Unfortunately the bacteria responsible for the problem can develop a resistance to antibiotics and the ear infections become chronic for some children. You can make some simple and safe aromatherapy ear drops to protect and heal little ears.

> 10 drops tea tree essential oil
> 10 drops blue chamomile essential oil
> 10 drops lavender essential oil
> 30 ml (1 ounce) olive oil

Combine the oils in a 30 ml (1 ounce) eyedropper bottle and shake to mix.

To use: During cold and flu season, using an eyedropper or pipette, administer one to three drops in each ear daily. If the child has a cold or congestion, or if there is an existing ear infection, you can add a mashed fresh clove of garlic to the oil mixture and then filter or strain to increase its healing action.

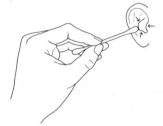

A child's ear infection can be treated by gently applying chamomile oil around the outer edge of the ear canal with a cotton swab.

CHILDREN'S MASSAGE OIL FOR COLDS, ACHES, AND PAINS

10 drops geranium essential oil
5 drop sandalwood essential oil
5 drops MQV essential oil
60 ml (2 ounces) almond or apricot oil

Mix and store in a small dark glass bottle.

To use: When your child is bedridden with a cold or flu, ease aches and pains with a healing and soothing massage with this oil.

BRONCHITIS FORMULA FOR BABIES AND CHILDREN

The congestion associated with bronchitis can make for some sleepless nights for both child and parent. For a more restful night, try one of these blends.

Formula 1

Mix 2 drops each of hyssop and lavender oil into a piece of softened cocoa butter, about the size of the tip of your little finger. Mold the butter into a little suppository and place it on wax paper in the refrigerator to firm up.

To use: At bedtime, to relieve bronchial congestion during the night, gently insert the suppository into the child's rectum.

Formula 2

Blend together 5 ml (1 teaspoon) each of *Eucalyptus radiata* and lavender in a diffuser.

To use: Run diffuser for two to four hours at night or all night on a low setting.

Formula 3

Make a massage oil with 5 drops of *Eucalyptus radiata* and 5 drops of lavender added to 30 ml (1 ounce) of almond oil.

To use: Rub into the chest and back areas.

Diarrhea Formula

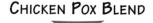

    5 drops neroli essential oil
    30 ml (1 ounce) carrier oil

Combine oils in small dark glass bottle.
To use: Massage on the tummy to relieve cramping and help the gut return to normal function.

Chicken Pox Blend

    5 drops tea tree essential oil
    1 drop peppermint essential oil
    30 ml (1 ounce) milk

For a soothing and antiseptic chicken pox treatment, mix the tea tree and peppermint in milk and stir into a warm bath.

Sadness Soother

Young children can have emotional upsets, mainly as a result of disappointments and hurt feelings.

    10 drops ylang ylang essential oil
    5 drops rose essential oil
    5 drops marjoram essential oil
    60 ml (2 ounces) almond or apricot oil

Mix and store in a small dark glass bottle.
To use: When a child is dealing with sadness or hurt feelings, a massage with this blend can soothe emotional pain.

POX HEALER

When the lesions of chicken pox have dried and begun to heal, mix equal parts of rose hip seed oil and everlasting essential oil, and dab onto the pox marks with a cotton swab to promote healing and prevent pox scars.

GRIEF BLEND

We all must deal with grief in our lives, but children can be hit particularly hard. Even the loss of a favored pet can cause intense grief for small children, and they may need help expressing their pain.

> 5 drops mandarin essential oil
> 5 drops peppermint essential oil
> 5 drops bergamot essential oil
> 5 drops neroli essential oil
> 60 ml (2 ounces) almond or apricot oil

Mix and store in a small dark glass bottle.

To use: A massage with this blend can be helpful to a child who is grieving over a loss in life.

A BLEND FOR THE VICTIM OF ABUSE OR NEGLECT

Baby animals that are left untouched suffer from weakened immune systems, and show retarded emotional and social development. Neglected and abused children show similar symptoms. These children sometimes have a very difficult time being touched. Very gentle massage can help such children regain trust.

> 10 drops lavender essential oil
> 5 drops geranium essential oil
> 5 drops sandalwood essential oil
> 60 ml (2 ounces) almond or apricot oil

Mix and store in a small dark glass bottle.

To use: A massage with this blend would be healing to an emotionally injured child.

AROMATHERAPY FOR TEENAGERS

The teen years are probably the first really difficult period in life. Adolescence brings hormonal changes, which radically affect the personality. The strange new appearance of body hair, odors, pimples, and skin rashes can be unsettling for this age group. Teens are faced with many new challenges — from peers to school and family. Society in general often looks upon teens with a somewhat jaded view. The natural rebellion that surges up inside an individual toward both parental and societal restrictions creates an alienation within many youths. Some teens adhere to the rules and some fight the rules. Both choices carry their own stress.

Developing a healthy lifestyle and learning how to treat their bodies with care and respect are important tasks for teens. The stress of the adolescent years, when added to a nutritionally inadequate diet and overconsumption of junk food and sugars, can undermine a teenager's physical and emotional health.

Aromatherapy offers teens a unique opportunity to honor themselves and control their destiny with a naturally supported healthy lifestyle. My young aromatherapy students and clients have ranged in age from newborn through the teen years. I owe special thanks to Cassandra, Sky, Crystal, Russell, Samuel, and Silas for many valuable insights.

Hygiene

Teenagers are the worst victims of vanity. The rapid changes they are experiencing, combined with an exaggerated awareness of the opposite sex, often contribute to a distorted self-image. Teens are extremely critical of one another, and view their own flaws as if through a magnifying lens. They can be horrified by their own body odor or greasy hair, and a pimple can precipitate a major emotional crisis.

IMPORTANT OILS FOR TEENS

Basil
Bergamot
Cinnamon
Clary sage
Clove
Coriander
Eucalyptus
Jasmine
Juniper
Lavender
Lemon
Lemongrass
Mandarin
Orange
Patchouli
Peppermint
Rosemary
Sweet thyme
Tea tree
Ylang ylang

Hair Formulas

Try any of these aromatherapy treatments for hair:

- A few drops of lemongrass and rosemary oils added to a bottle of ordinary shampoo will make a balancing and conditioning hair treatment.
- Two to 3 drops of lemon oil in a cup (235 ml) of warm water makes an effective final rinse for oily hair.
- Two to 3 drops of rosemary oil in a cup (235 ml) of warm water makes an effective final rinse for dry hair.
- Two drops of rosemary oil sprinkled directly on the hairbrush will tame unruly hair and minimize breakage by helping tangles brush out easily.

Body Odor Blend

A very effective deodorant dusting powder can be made with dry white clay.

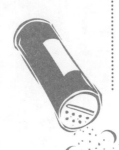

```
  5  drops coriander essential oil
 15  drops lavender essential oil
225  g (8 ounces) white clay
```

Stir the oils into the clay and store in an airtight widemouthed jar.
To use: Dust on after bathing to control body odor.

ATHLETE'S FOOT FORMULA

The communal showers at schools and gymnasiums are a breeding ground for fungal infections. Athlete's foot can be an itchy nuisance, but if left untreated it can become chronic and painful. You can make a foot powder that combats fungus well as it dries out the skin.

    2 drops thyme essential oil
    5 drops rosemary essential oil
    2 drops tagetes or savory essential oil
  225 g (8 ounces) white clay

Stir the oils into the clay and store in an airtight jar.
To use: Dust onto feet after showering, especially between the toes. Wear absorbent cotton athletic socks and change them often.

TATTOO AND PIERCING SOOTHER

Tattoos and body piercing present a danger from infection. Hygiene is of the utmost importance until the site has thoroughly healed. This antiseptic formula will soothe the skin and help the site heal quickly.

   30 ml (1 ounce) aloe vera gel
    5 drops tea tree essential oil
   10 drops lavender essential oil
    2 drops blue chamomile essential oil

Put the aloe vera gel into a small plastic squeeze bottle, add the oils, and shake to blend.
To use: Squeeze a dab of this gel directly onto the tattoo or piercing site periodically throughout the day until the wound has healed.

Teenage Acne

The scourge of the teenage years, acne is often brought on by the hormonal changes associated with puberty, and exacerbated by stresses that are virtually built into a teenager's life. If left untreated, its victims are often scarred for life, both physically and emotionally. Fortunately, acne often responds well to a holistic approach.

Oral Acne Remedies. Tea tree is a remarkable oil that has proven effective for treating acne, as well as numerous other problems that plague teens. Before resorting to a course of oral antibiotics, a teen who is troubled with chronic acne would be well advised to try tea tree. A daily drop of tea tree oil applied directly on the back of the tongue will have a mild antibiotic action, and should show favorable results within one to two weeks.

The presence of bacteria on the surface of the skin is natural, but when those bacteria invade the open lesions of acne, small infections occur and the severity of the outbreak is increased. Essence of eucalyptus taken internally will have an antiseptic effect. Two drops, dissolved in honey and mixed in 1 cup (235 ml) of water, can be taken daily without harm.

The thickening and scarring of the acne process inhibits normal sloughing and cellular regeneration, and the complexion becomes congested with unshed toxins. Two drops of peppermint oil drunk once a day in a cup (235 ml) of water will have a detoxifying effect.

Topical Acne Remedies. To make a healing rinse for inflamed acne, add 2 drops of myrrh and 10 drops each of lavender and clary sage to 4 ounces (120 ml) of aromatic vinegar. Combine the ingredients in a clean bottle and shake to blend. After cleansing the face, soak a cotton ball with this vinegar rinse and blot the face all over generously.

FIGHT ACNE THROUGH DIET

Avoid excess sugar, caffeine, and carbonated drinks. Substitute herb teas, such as chamomile, yarrow, burdock root, and plantain. Take vitamin B_6 supplements and eat plenty of foods that are rich in minerals, including parsley, tomatoes, watercress, radishes, and wheat germ.

CLAY MASKS

Clay is a totally benevolent healing substance that absorbs toxins, tightens pores, and heals many skin eruptions. Clay masks blended with specific essential oils and hydrosols are a highly effective treatment for teens with acned skin, and also for occasional breakouts.

Drying Mask

The rose clay in this mask is most effective for oily and acne skin.

45	ml	(3 tablespoons) rose clay
60–75	ml	(4 to 5 tablespoons) distilled water or rose hydrosol
3	drops	*Eucalyptus radiata* essential oil
2	drops	melissa or lemon essential oil

Cleansing Mask

This recipe makes a cleansing and balancing mask for all skin types.

45	ml	(3 tablespoons) green clay
60–75	ml	(4 to 5 tablespoons) distilled water or lavender hydrosol
3	drops	tea tree essential oil
2	drops	spike lavender or neroli essential oil

For either recipe: Measure clay into a ceramic bowl. Using a wooden paddle or chopstick, stir in the water or hydrosol to form a soft paste. Add the essential oils and mix thoroughly.

To use: Apply clay in a thin layer all over the face, avoiding the tender skin around your eyes. Leave clay on until dry, then wash off with a washcloth and warm water. For an exfoliating treatment, scrub the dry clay off with your fingertips or a dry washcloth.

TIPS ON CLAY MASKS

- Each recipe will make enough paste for several treatments. Store the excess in an airtight glass or ceramic container.
- Apply mask up to three times a week. More frequent use of clay masks is not recommended.

Low Self-Esteem

The rapid changes of adolescence can be destabilizing to even the most confident child. Assertive little girls often become shy teenagers, and bright and friendly little boys often withdraw into a surly, uncommunicative adolescence. Most teens survive the difficult period with their original personalities intact, but low self-esteem during these years can make for a lonely and distressing adolescence.

A teen can, periodically throughout the day, inhale the scent of rose or palmarosa directly from the bottle to help restore perspective, and reduce harsh self-criticism. A few drops of either oil massaged directly onto the stomach, legs, and arms following the bath can also have a positive effect on self-esteem.

Depression

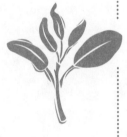

Dealing with parents, teachers, and friends is often difficult for teens. Coping with grades, setting goals, and managing a social life can be overwhelming. It's a sad statistic that teens suffer from severe depression and are subject to suicidal thoughts more often than any other age group. Frequent inhalations of clary sage, jasmine, or patchouli — or all three mixed together — can effectively dispel the most common depressive thoughts in just a few minutes.

Energy Fluctuations

Exhaustion can be a major contributing factor to emotional and physical problems. Teenagers have a tendency to overextend themselves, and often don't recognize their need for rest. What appears to be boundless energy can in reality be overstimulation of the adrenal system. Such a condition, if sustained for too long, can result in adrenal fatigue and a weakened immune system. Adrenal fatigue is best dealt with by taking frequent naps. Meditating also helps focus

ESSENTIAL OILS TO DEAL WITH STRESS

Stress	Essential Oils
Anger, to soothe	Chamomile, ylang ylang
Anger, unexpressed	Rosemary
Mental stress	Basil, citrus oils, neroli
Emotional stress	Sandalwood, lavender
PMS	Clary sage
Test anxiety	Mandarin, orange, lemongrass
Computer stress	Basil, mugwort

energy and restore exhausted adrenal systems. Running a diffuser with clary sage, bergamot, clove, and jasmine during meditation, naps, or quiet time will also support and restore a healthy adrenal system.

Common Colds and Flu

When teens get run down, they are particularly susceptible to colds, flus, and other viral illnesses. Fortunately, they are resilient and usually recover quickly. When everything hurts and a teen's got the blues, a nice hot soaking bath can bring comfort.

TEEN PICK-ME-UP

5 drops eucalyptus essential oil
5 drops geranium essential oil
5 drops sandalwood essential oil
5 drops juniper essential oil
120 ml (4 ounces) milk

Stir the oils into the milk and disperse in a hot bath. Soak until the water turns tepid.

First Periods and Menstrual Distress

Sometimes teenagers suffer exaggerated menstrual distress with their first few periods. The severity of symptoms usually decreases after several months, although there are those women who suffer through painful periods throughout their reproductive life. Rose oil exerts a considerable influence on the female organs. It is believed to regulate hormone levels, making it invaluable for supporting a healthy menstrual cycle. You can inhale the scent of rose oil directly from the bottle or mix 1 or 2 drops of rose oil with 1 ounce (30 ml) of almond oil and massage onto the stomach, over the ovaries, or onto the lower back.

Emmenagogues. Young girls often exhibit symptoms of menstrual cycling for months before they actually begin having periods. These symptoms can include bloating, cramping, and diarrhea, as well as headache, fatigue, and depression. It is appropriate to treat such symptoms as you would menstrual distress. The formula listed above will surely provide some relief. If your teen seems poised at the brink of puberty and is suffering what might be described as prolonged premenstrual syndrome, the administration of an emmenagogue may ease her discomfort by encouraging the onset of menstruation.

Choose one or two essential oils from the emmenagogue list in the box at left and mix a total of 2 to 3 drops into 1 ounce (30 ml) of almond oil. Massage onto the stomach, over the ovaries, or onto the lower back.

Vaginal Infections

The *Candida albicans* organism is present in all of us and causes no problems when it remains at a healthy level. When it grows beyond a healthy level, however, it can cause problems. The most common manifestation of candida overgrowth is what we call a

---

EMMENAGOGUE OILS

An emmenagogue encourages menstruation. Essential oils that have an emmenagogue action are:

Basil

Clary sage

Fennel

Juniper

Marjoram

Myrrh

Peppermint

Rose

Rosemary

vaginal yeast infection. The overgrowth can be due to a number of factors, including overuse of antibiotics, overconsumption of sugar, and overexposure to stress. The condition comes on fast and can make a woman miserable with its itching, irritation, and discharge. A yeast infection can be simply and effectively treated with essential oils.

YEAST INFECTION BOLUS BLEND

Boluses are female vaginal suppositories, also called ovules, that are used to treat vaginal infections. You can easily make your own with a cocoa butter base.

60 g (2 ounces) cocoa butter
30 g (1 ounce) white clay
 4 drops cocoa butter essential oil
 4 drops tea tree essential oil
 5 drops lavender essential oil

1. Melt the cocoa butter over low heat.
2. Remove from heat and add the clay and essential oils.
3. Chill the mixture until the cocoa butter just begins to harden, then form into boluses, about the size and shape of the tip of your little finger, and place them on a sheet of wax paper in the refrigerator.
4. When the boluses have hardened, store them in an airtight glass container in the refrigerator.
To use: To treat a yeast infection or other vaginal irritation, insert one bolus vaginally each night before bed. Treatment can be safely continued for one to two weeks.

Yeast Infection Sponge Blend

2 drops lavender essential oil
2 drops tea tree essential oil
2 drops myrrh essential oil

You will need a small, sterile cosmetic sponge. You can purchase a "silk," or natural sponge, from your druggist that will work quite well. Tie a length of dental floss to the sponge, leaving a 4-inch (10 cm) "tail" for convenient retrieval. (See page 103.)

Disperse the essential oils into a cup (235 ml) of warm water and immerse the sponge. Gently squeeze out the excess moisture — so it is not dripping — and insert the sponge into the vagina, leaving it overnight. You can wear a sanitary pad for security.

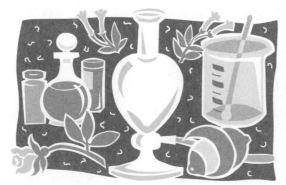

Aromatherapy for Pregnancy and Menopause

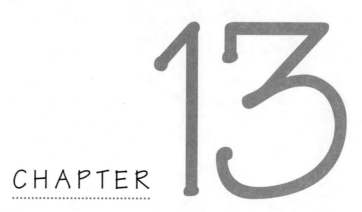

CHAPTER 13

Pregnancy is a special time in a woman's life. It is a time when a woman pays close attention to her body. As her concern for her growing baby expands, her old attitudes toward self-care are revisited and often revised. During pregnancy, most women experience a heightened sense of smell. Familiar foods and cosmetics elicit unfamiliar responses. If this is your first pregnancy, appreciate that it is a unique time in your life. Take the opportunity to learn as much as you can about pregnancy. Use the experience to get to know your body. I hope your experience with pregnancy will be enjoyable and memorable.

Aromatherapy has specific applications that can enhance your experience of pregnancy. Knowing which essential oils to use and which to avoid is very important.

AROMATHERAPY DURING PREGNANCY

An average pregnancy is considered to take 40 weeks to reach full term. This period is split up into three trimesters.

The first trimester is an especially important time, when the risk of injury to the unborn is great. During this period the baby's organs are just developing and are vulnerable to serious damage from exposure to toxins, drugs, and other influential chemicals. A pregnant woman's heightened sense of smell may be Mother Nature's way of helping her avoid things that could do harm to her or her baby.

There are some oils that should be avoided during the early months of pregnancy (see list at right). They may, however, be safely used during the second and third trimesters for very specific applications.

Morning Sickness

Morning sickness is often one of the first signs of pregnancy. It can range in severity from a slight queasiness upon awakening in the morning to severe nausea and vomiting throughout the day. While the queasiness may be just a mild nuisance, the more severe forms of morning sickness can cause the mother to become dehydrated and undernourished, and can undermine the health of mother and baby. Here are a few aromatic remedies for morning sickness:

◆ One drop of peppermint oil (no more!) taken in a glass of honey water first thing in the morning is very calming to the stomach. Dill (or cinnamon in the second trimester) can be substituted for the peppermint with a similar effect.

◆ If nausea is so severe that fluids aren't being retained, an inhalation is indicated. Place a few drops of either peppermint, dill, or cinnamon on a cotton ball and keep it with you in an airtight vial. Periodically inhale the scent throughout the day.

Stretch Marks

Stretch marks can be prevented with a twice-daily massage throughout your pregnancy with one of these formulas. Rub the blend over the skin of the abdomen, breasts, and hips to increase elasticity and help preserve the skin's normal texture.

STRETCH MARK CREAM

Cocoa butter is a wonderful emollient that melts on contact with the skin in warm weather. If you live in a cold climate and find that this cocoa butter base sets up too hard, making it difficult to apply, you can substitute sesame, olive, or almond oil for the cocoa butter.

    30 ml (1 ounce) cocoa butter
     4 drops jasmine essential oil
    12 drops mandarin essential oil

Melt the cocoa butter and stir in the essential oils. Store in a wide-mouthed jar.

OILS TO AVOID

Avoid these oils during the first trimester:

Aniseed	Cinnamon
Basil	Clary sage
Bitter	Clove
almond	Fennel
Calamus	Hyssop
Camphor	Juniper
Caraway	Marjoram
Cedarwood	Myrrh

Avoid these oils throughout the entire pregnancy:

Mugwort	Sassafras
Myrrh	Savory
Nutmeg	Tansy
Oregano	Thuja
Pennyroyal	Thyme
Rosemary	Wintergreen
Rue	Wormwood
Sage	

STRETCH MARK OIL

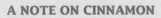

30 ml (1 ounce) carrier oil
4 drops lavender essential oil
4 drops chamomile essential oil
4 drops neroli essential oil
2 drops rose essential oil

For this blend, I recommend a mixture of almond and wheat germ oils for your carrier. Aim for approximately 90 percent almond oil to 10 percent wheat germ oil. Start by measuring 27 ml (just under 1 ounce) of almond oil, then add 3 ml wheat germ oil to equal 30 ml (1 ounce). Blend in the essential oils.

To use: Apply twice daily to the stomach area, breasts, and hips.

Hemorrhoids

Hemorrhoids are congested veins around the rectum and anus. They are caused, or aggravated, by the pelvic congestion of pregnancy. To prevent and ease hemorrhoids, avoid constipation. Eat plenty of fiber and include psyllium seed in your diet.

Twenty drops of cypress oil dispersed in your bathwater will relieve hemorrhoid pressure. The cypress has a vasoconstricting action that will tighten tissue and shrink painful hemorrhoids.

HEMORRHOID GEL

4 drops cypress essential oil
2 drops geranium essential oil
2 drops Roman chamomile essential oil
30 ml (1 ounce) aloe vera gel

Blend the essential oils into the aloe vera gel.

A NOTE ON CINNAMON
Although cinnamon is considered an unsafe oil during the first trimester, 1 drop diluted in a soluble solution such as olive oil or honey can be safely ingested to control morning sickness.

To use: Apply as a compress to relieve pain and swelling of hemorrhoids. Apply with a sterile cotton cloth or on a sanitary napkin.

Varicose Veins

Varicose veins are caused by congestion and poor circulation through the pelvic area. Many women develop them during pregnancy. The legs are affected, usually around the knee and ankle areas.

LEG MASSAGE OIL

Make a simple lotion to relieve restless legs and leg pain and to reduce and prevent varicose veins.

    10 drops cypress essential oil
     5 drops lemon essential oil
    60 ml (2 ounces) carrier oil

Blend the essential oils into the carrier oil.
To use: Massage the legs, working from the ankles toward the groin, and stroking in the direction of the heart.

LEG BATH OIL

    10 drops lavender essential oil
     5 drops cypress essential oil
    90 ml (3 ounces) milk

Blend the oils into the milk.
To use: Disperse in a *warm* bath (a hot bath will aggravate varicose veins). You can make the application extra effective by elevating your feet as high as possible while you soak.

EASING VARICOSE VEINS

Elevating your feet above your heart for 10 minutes every day is an excellent practice that will prevent the development of varicose veins as well as ease the severity of existing ones.

Edema

Edema is an abnormal retention of fluids. Most pregnant women experience minor edema as a swelling of the hands, feet, and ankles. Minor edema is usually not threatening to the health of mother or baby, but it can be a signal that the kidneys are struggling. Elevating the feet can help reduce swelling. Dietary remedies include drinking plenty of water and natural fruit juices, and avoiding overconsumption of salts or sugars.

WATERY LEGS MASSAGE OIL BLEND

10 drops lavender essential oil   10 drops lemon essential oil
4 drops geranium essential oil   60 ml (2 ounces) almond oil
4 drops cypress essential oil

Blend the essential oils into the almond oil and mix well.
To use: Massage the legs, working from the ankles toward the groin, and stroking in the direction of the heart.

Back Pain

Back pain is common during the later stages of pregnancy, and massage with essential oils can bring a wonderful relief. As the body is changing and stretching, the added body weight puts strain on the muscles. Hormonal changes cause the ligaments around the spine and pelvic to soften.

PRENATAL MASSAGE OIL

5 drops sandalwood essential oil   5 drops ylang ylang
5 drops eucalyptus essential oil   essential oil
5 drops mandarin essential oil   30 ml (1 ounce) almond oil

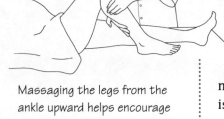

Massaging the legs from the ankle upward helps encourage circulation and prevent bloating during pregnancy.

Combine all oils and mix well.

To use: Pain and discomfort can be minimized or erased by a gentle massage with this blend.

PRENATAL BATH BLEND

An aromatic bath can ease back pain and general spinal stress.

     5 drops chamomile essential oil
    12 drops lavender essential oil
     2 drops neroli essential oil

To use: Disperse the essential oils into a warm bath and soak. This blend will also ease the pain of ligament stretching in the groin area and help prevent constipation.

Indigestion and Heartburn

As the baby grows bigger it pushes on the stomach, causing indigestion and heartburn. Foods that were previously tolerated well can begin to cause problems. It is a good idea to avoid spicy foods, fatty foods, and overeating in general during the third trimester.

HEARTBURN MASSAGE OIL

     6 drops mandarin essential oil
     3 drops neroli essential oil
     6 drops sandalwood essential oil
    30 ml (1 ounce) almond oil

Blend the essential oils in the almond oil and mix well.

To use: Massage over the stomach and liver area to relieve painful indigestion or heartburn.

A SIMPLE AROMA STOMACH REMEDY

Dissolve 1 drop of sandalwood in 1 cup (235 ml) of honey water, a tablespoon of aloe vera gel, or a solubol solution. Sandalwood has a slightly bitter taste and the sweetness of the solubol solution makes it more palatable. Taken this way at night, sandalwood will also help you sleep.

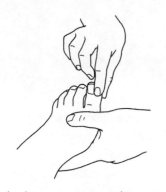

Applying pressure to this point alongside the big toe can help relieve labor pains.

PREPARATION FOR LABOR

Toward the end of pregnancy, in the eighth month, you can begin to use one or two of the forbidden oils such as clary sage and fennel. These two are excellent for strengthening the womb and stimulating milk production.

One or 2 drops of either clary or fennel oil can now be added to stretch mark oil for local application. In the last weeks of pregnancy, one drop of fennel taken in a cup (235 ml) of hot honey water will stimulate estrogen and help prepare the body for producing adequate breast milk.

Many midwives routinely use aromatherapy to ease labor and facilitate childbirth. Specific oils are chosen for their calming, energizing, and uplifting effects, as well as for their delicious scents. Massage is a natural way to support and nurture the laboring woman, and the addition of aromatherapy enhances the positive effect.

Besides the lower back, shoulders, and legs, the reflex corresponding to the solar plexus located on the sole of the foot is massaged to minimize stress during birthing. There is also a pressure point located alongside the large toenail, which provides a degree of relief from the most intense labor pains.

Prepare massage oils that will be used during labor in advance. To prepare any of the following blends, fill a 1-ounce (30 ml) bottle with almond oil, leaving a little room at the top. Add the essential oils, cap, and shake.

LABOR BLEND RECIPES

Formula 1

10 drops lavender essential oil

2 drops rose essential oil

5 drops clary sage essential oil

30 ml (1 ounce) almond oil

Formula 2

10 drops lavender essential oil

6 drops palmarosa
essential oil

4 drops sweet thyme
essential oil

30 ml (1 ounce) almond oil

Formula 3

10 drops lavender essential oil

2 drops rose essential oil

5 drops ylang ylang
essential oil

30 ml (1 ounce) almond oil

Formula 4

5 drops geranium essential oil

3 drops Roman chamomile
essential oil

6 drops palmarosa
essential oil

30 ml (1 ounce) almond oil

Formula 5

6 drops mandarin essential oil

3 drops neroli essential oil

6 drops palmarosa
essential oil

30 ml (1 ounce) almond oil

POSTNATAL CARE

If the perineum has been cut — an episiotomy — and there are
stitches, they can be healed quickly with essential oil skin washes.
Cypress tightens the tissue, and lavender soothes and helps heal the
site of the episiotomy. Everlasting decreases scarring from surgery
or stiches.

POSTNATAL SKIN SOOTHER

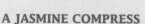

5 drops lavender essential oil

3 drops cypress essential oil

2 drops everlasting essential oil

To use: Disperse the essential oils into a basin of hot water. Wet a
clean washcloth in the basin, wring it out to make a warm compress, and place it over the episiotomy site.

A JASMINE COMPRESS

Many midwives use jas-
mine in a compress on
the lower abdomen to
help expel the placenta.
Disperse 5 drops of jas-
mine into a basin of hot
water. Wet a clean towel
in the basin, wring it
out, and place the warm,
wet towel over the
abdomen following birth.

Postpartum Depression

After giving birth, some women experience a period of depression. This depression can range from a slight letdown after the exhilarating experience of labor and delivery to a severe and acute depression that renders a mother incapable of caring for, and bonding with, her newborn. Acute postpartum depression is a serious problem and can be life threatening. A new mother who appears listless or distraught should never be left alone to care for her infant. The emotional and physical support of other women is crucial, and medical intervention is indicated in severe cases.

Some essential oils that are helpful in relieving mild postpartum depression are bergamot, cinnamon, clary sage, clove, geranium, grapefruit, jasmine, neroli, orange, petitgrain, and rose. Place a drop or two of any of these oils on a handkerchief or tissue and inhale the scent periodically throughout the day.

LACTATION MASSAGE BLEND

To promote lactation, massage breasts with either of these blends.

Formula 1

> 10 drops fennel essential oil
> 5 drops lemongrass essential oil
> 60 ml (2 ounces) carrier oil

Formula 2

> 6 drops fennel essential oil
> 6 drops geranium essential oil
> 60 ml (2 ounces) carrier oil

Breast Care Tips

Aromatherapy oils can help ease sensitive breasts during pregnancy and following birth.

♦ To treat sore and cracked nipples, add 1 drop of rose essential oil to 1 ounce (30 ml) of aloe vera gel. Apply sparingly to the distressed area.

♦ If the breasts become engorged, apply warm compresses of lavender and geranium. Disperse 2 to 3 drops of each essential oil into a basin of hot water. Wet a clean towel in the basin, wring it out to make a warm compress, and place it over the breasts.

♦ Mastitis (infection of the milk ducts in the breast) can be a very painful condition. With a newborn, it is important to keep the milk flowing through the breasts. Mastitis can be treated with the same compress used to treat engorgement. If fever is present, add a drop of peppermint for a cooling effect.

♦ When the time has come to wean your child, you can inhibit lactation by applying a sage compress to the breasts. Disperse 4 drops of sage oil into a basin of hot water. Wet a clean towel in the basin, wring it out to make a warm compress, and place it over the breasts.

♦ Soaking in a hot bath into which 4 drops of sage and 4 drops of geranium essential oil have been dispersed will also inhibit lactation.

AROMATHERAPY FOR MENOPAUSE

Too often, our modern culture treats menopause as a disease. Some women do experience this period as a turbulent time, but menopause is a natural stage in a woman's life and should be approached as the beginning of a new cycle rather than the end of youth. Menopause can actually mark the beginning of the most powerful and productive time of a woman's life. In Thailand a woman enters menopause with a celebration, announcing to friends and family that she has grown beyond her childbearing years. In many primitive societies a post-menopausal woman enjoys an elevated status. She often assumes the role of a shaman or healer within her tribe. If you are approaching or entering this cycle of your life, learn about women who have done well and survived menopause in a strong way.

By the time a woman is 45, most of her ovarian follicles have ripened and ovulated, leaving just a few to secrete estrogen and progesterone. Over the next few years these too will most likely be used up, and her two ovaries will no longer function as active glands. Her production of feminizing hormones will virtually cease. Ideally these changes occur gradually and, as her monthly cycles come to an end, a woman's body adjusts to the change in its hormonal environment. Many women, however, experience a sudden onset of menopause following a hysterectomy or other gynecological surgery, ovarian or uterine cancer, or chemotherapy treatment for breast or other cancers.

Treating Common Symptoms

There are a variety of unpleasant side effects of the hormonal imbalances that are common to this stage of a woman's life. She may suffer from hot flashes, heat rashes, night sweats, and insomnia. Her symptoms may include irritability, fatigue, anxiety, and depression. She may develop vaginal atrophy and dryness, heart disease, and osteoporosis. Some women begin to experience panic attacks and feel as if they are dying. Others want to, and even contemplate suicide.

Hormone replacement therapy is often prescribed to relieve such unpleasant symptoms and to reduce the health risks associated with menopause. But most women experience only a few of these symptoms, and these for only a brief period. The radical hormonal adjustments of a medically induced menopause, however, can cause multiple and acute symptoms, complicating recovery from what was most likely a difficult and unsettling event in a woman's life. Routine hormone replacement therapy is not recommended for women with a family history of breast, uterine, or ovarian cancer, liver disease, thrombosis, fibrocystic breasts, migraines, or endometriosis. Moreover, many women are now turning to alternative therapies and choosing to address menopause as a natural phase of their lives rather than as a malady requiring medical management.

Dietary Guidelines

To counteract menopausal symptoms, ensure your diet is rich in nutrients. Consume an abundance of clean water, fresh vegetables and juices, and whole grains. If they are not already a part of your diet, introduce soy products and sea vegetables. Now is a good time to add vitamin supplements to your health-maintenance program: antioxidants, B-complex vitamins, and especially vitamin E, which is in the membrane covering every cell in the body and is vital to life.

Avoid overconsumption of alcohol, caffeine, carbonated sodas, sugar, refined carbohydrates, and fatty foods. Besides being nutritionally deficient foods, they tax the immune system and deplete the body of crucial minerals. It is particularly important in midlife to get adequate minerals, especially zinc. Colloidal mineral supplements, derived from the clay of ancient seabeds, provide a broad range of these necessary minerals in an accessible form. Colloidal particles are so small that they can remain suspended in liquid or gas, but unlike dissolved particles, they retain their whole form.

Natural Remedies

Dioscorea villosa, or wild yam root, rediscovered in the 1980s, has actually been used to treat menopausal discomforts for centuries. According to the Chinese pharmacopoeia, shu-yu (wild yam) is tonic, restorative, and cooling; it benefits the spirit, brightens the intellect, and prolongs life.

The primary active ingredient of the wild yam is thought to be diosgenin, which acts much like a natural progesterone, performing as an adaptogen, or balancer in the body. Formulated into a skin cream, the active ingredients are absorbed transdermally, which makes the wild yam an excellent complement to aromatherapy remedies. There are many different wild yam creams commercially available. Some are formulated with herbs and essential oils for a synergistic effect. If you choose to use a wild yam cream to alleviate menopausal discomforts, you can add lavender, geranium, angelica, spikenard, fennel, sage, clary sage, or melissa. These oils are considered prehormones and phytoestrogens. They help balance the hormones and, through their own actions, can alleviate menopausal discomforts.

Menopause Blends

The following formulas address specific problems that are often associated with either menopause or premenstrual syndrome. These blends can be mixed into a massage or body oil, or added to a bath. To make a bath solution, dissolve the essential oils in 2 ounces (60 ml) of solubol or milk before adding to the bath. For a body or massage oil, mix the essential oils into ⅔ ounce (20 ml) of either apricot or macadamia nut oil to which you have added ⅓ ounce (10 ml) of either borage, evening primrose, or rose hip seed oil.

PREMENSTRUAL DISTRESS FORMULA

This is an excellent blend for treating unpleasant premenstrual or premenopausal symptoms.

5 drops geranium essential oil
2 drops sage essential oil
10 drops clary sage essential oil
2 drops angelica essential oil

CAUTION
This blend should not be used during pregnancy or lactation because of the sage.

Yin-Yang Balance

This blend, which stimulates and balances masculine energy, is helpful in situations in which estrogen is dominant.

5 drops *Pinus maritima* essential oil
3 drops *Pinus siberian* essential oil
2 drops angelica essential oil

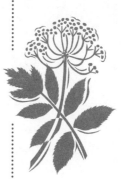

Menopause Comforter

A comforting blend to use during a rough time. Use this blend to treat stress or insomnia.

4 drops Roman chamomile essential oil
4 drops spike lavender essential oil
4 drops lavender essential oil
2 drops clary sage essential oil

Uplifting Blend

Use this uplifting blend during times of hormonal imbalance or depression.

3 drops bergamot essential oil
2 drops myrrh essential oil
2 drops ylang ylang essential oil
4 drops fennel essential oil
4 drops geranium essential oil

WARMING BLEND

This warming blend is energizing to the libido.

4 drops black pepper essential oil
4 drops cedarwood essential oil
3 drops ylang ylang essential oil
3 drops sandalwood essential oil

All of these blends will enhance a woman's health and can be used throughout the life cycle, but they are particularly beneficial during midlife.

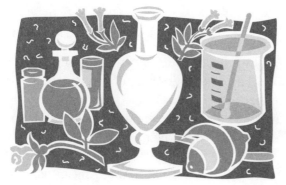

Men and
Aromatherapy

Aromatherapy is not just for women. Men are also highly influenced by scent, and aromatherapy offers them an effective means of directing their emotional and physical energy as well as managing their general health. Over the years, many of my most enthusiastic students have been men. Men love the idea of using natural aromas to calm, stimulate, and regulate the human body. This section speaks directly to you gentlemen and your particular needs.

ESSENTIAL OILS FOR MEN

Many essential oils specifically evoke masculine or feminine energy (see box at left). Although these are considered the more masculine oils, they are truly balancing and helpful to men wishing to connect with their sensual and emotional nature. As my friend Steve explains, "Aromatherapy helps to get me in touch with my olfactory sense, one of the senses I have pretty much taken for granted. It helps me to feel grounded. By that I mean using oils helps me to come into my body and *feel* myself more."

A customer named Brian says it more simply: "I enjoy smelling different oils, applying them, and honoring myself."

SKIN CARE FOR MEN

Aftershave lotions are meant to be antiseptic — to prevent the infection of small razor nicks — as well as bracing and clarifying. Many men find commercial aftershave products irritate their skin, being too drying and abrasive. This aftershave gel will clarify the complexion and soothe and protect irritated skin.

MANLY SCENTS

Bay laurel
Cedar
Cistus
Clary sage
Clove
Jasmine
Juniper
Lavender
Lime
Oregano
Pine
Rosemary
Sandalwood
Savory
Tea tree
Thyme
Vetiver

AFTERSHAVE GEL

10 drops lavender essential oil
4 drops neroli essential oil
2 drops cistus essential oil
120 ml (4 ounces) aloe vera gel

Mix and store in a 120 ml (4 ounce) dark glass bottle. You can keep a small amount in a small plastic bottle for dispensing.

HAPPY FEET

Much used and much abused are our poor feet. Imprisoned in socks and shoes most of their lives, they deserve some extra care and attention.

ATHLETE'S FOOT POWDER

12 drops lavender essential oil
6 drops tea tree essential oil
2 drops savory essential oil
60 g (2 ounces) white clay

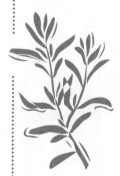

Combine the essential oils with the clay powder in a widemouthed jar. Stir thoroughly.

To use: Apply this powder on bare feet to soothe and heal the burning itch of athlete's foot. Sprinkle the powder in your shoes to ward off the unfriendly fungus.

ANTIFUNGAL NAIL OIL

Nail fungus is a common problem for men, causing their toenails to thicken and turn yellow.

5 drops tea tree essential oil	2 drops savory essential oil
2 drops cinnamon essential oil	15 ml (1 tablespoon) neem oil

Mix the ingredients in a 30 ml (1 ounce) bottle and shake well.
To use: Apply around and under the nail bed two to three times a day to treat fungus and promote healthy, normal nail growth.

FOOT OIL

For moisturizing dry feet.

6 drops myrrh essential oil	2 drops patchouli essential oil
10 drops sandalwood essential oil	30 ml (1 ounce) peanut oil
	30 ml (1 ounce) olive oil

Blend all ingredients in a 60 ml (2 ounce) bottle.
To use: Massage into the feet in the evening after a shower or bath.

FOOT LOTION

Great for invigorating hot, tired feet, this blend is refreshing and energizing for feet that still have a long way to go.

5 drops peppermint essential oil
60 ml (2 ounces) unscented lotion

Combine ingredients in a 60 ml (2 ounce) bottle.

ATHLETIC RUBS

Athletes know the value of a good muscle liniment. They look for analgesic action to relieve muscle aches and pains, along with heating or cooling action. These formulas are simple to make and can be used before or after workouts. Before going out in cold weather, use a warming oil on your legs to avoid strains. After a vigorous workout, use calming massage oils to relax the muscles and release built-up lactic acids.

STIMULATING SPORTS MASSAGE OIL

3 drops birch essential oil
6 drops pine essential oil
6 drops lemon essential oil
4 drops spruce essential oil
6 drops rosemary essential oil
60 ml (2 ounces) almond oil

Mix the ingredients in a 60 ml (2 ounce) bottle and shake well.
To use: Massage onto sore, achy muscles.

CALMING SPORTS MASSAGE OIL

3 drops birch essential oil
6 drops pine essential oil
6 drops eucalyptus essential oil
2 drops chamomile essential oil
60 ml (2 ounces) almond oil

Mix the ingredients in a 60 ml (2 ounce) bottle and shake well.
To use: Massage onto stiff, tired muscles.

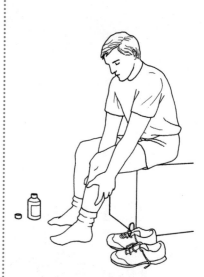

Applying massage oils after working out can help relieve sore muscles and prevent chronic aches.

REJUVENATING AND WARMING MASSAGE OIL

2 drops cinnamon essential oil

6 drops eucalyptus essential oil

6 drops camphor essential oil

4 drops clove essential oil

2 drops peppermint essential oil

12 drops lavender essential oil

6 drops orange essential oil

60 ml (2 ounces) almond oil

Mix the ingredients in a 60 ml (2 ounce) bottle and shake well.

To use: Massage onto sleepy, tight muscles. This is an excellent choice before cold-weather workouts.

FATIGUE BLEND

When you're feeling depleted, this blend will support the adrenals and restore vital energy.

6 drops cedarwood essential oil

4 drops bay laurel essential oil

4 drops spruce essential oil

60 ml (2 ounces) almond oil

Combine all oils in a 60 ml (2 ounce) bottle and mix well.

To use: Massage this blend on the legs and over the lower back and kidney area.

CAUTION

Cedar essential oil should not be used if you have high blood pressure.

EXHAUSTION BLEND

Exhaustion is beyond fatigue. Prolonged exhaustion will undermine good health. Where fatigue is a healthy response to physical exertion, exhaustion is a result of extreme stress. Both physical and emotional stress are usually components of exhaustion.

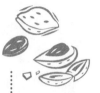

6 drops *Pinus pinaster* essential oil
6 drops *Pinus siberian* essential oil
6 drops mandarin petitgrain essential oil
2 drops savory essential oil
60 ml (2 ounces) almond oil

Mix the ingredients in a 60 ml (2 ounce) bottle and shake well.
To use: Massage over the whole body to support the adrenals and stimulate male hormone function.

RELAXING MASSAGE OIL BLEND

The following three formulas are excellent for general stress relief. They are calming, relaxing, and balancing to the male system.

Formula 1

6 drops marjoram essential oil
3 drops chamomile essential oil
10 drops lavender essential oil
3 drops sage essential oil
60 ml (2 ounces) almond oil

Formula 2

10 drops mandarin essential oil
2 drops jasmine essential oil
6 drops sandalwood essential oil
3 drops frankincense essential oil
60 ml (2 ounces) apricot oil

Formula 3

    10 drops bois de rose essential oil
     2 drops vetiver essential oil
     5 drops cedarwood essential oil
     3 drops frankincense essential oil
    60 ml (2 ounces) apricot oil

Mix all the ingredients in a 60 ml (2 ounce) bottle and shake well.

PROSTATE PROBLEMS

As men age, they often experience problems related to an enlarged prostate. The most common symptom is frequent urination, but urinary incontinence, degraded erectile function, and general malaise can occur in advanced stages.

INFLAMED PROSTATE RELIEVER

If his prostate becomes inflamed, a man may experience a painful burning sensation while urinating, or general abdominal pain and difficulty urinating. Massage with any of the prostate blends will provide relief, as will the following blend delivered rectally in a suppository.

    60 ml (2 ounces) cocoa butter
    10 drops geranium essential oil
     5 drops cypress essential oil
     2 drops peppermint essential oil

1. Melt the cocoa butter over low heat.
2. Remove from heat and add the essential oils.

3. Chill the mixture until the cocoa butter just begins to harden, then form suppositories about the size and shape of the tip of your little finger.

4. Place them on a sheet of wax paper in the refrigerator. When they have hardened, store them in an airtight glass container in the refrigerator.

To use: Insert at night to relieve symptoms of inflamed prostate.

French Prostate Massage Oil

In France, mastic *(Pistacia lentiscus)* is commonly used in a massage oil for decongesting the prostate. Mastic is a resin and a challenge to work with due to its extreme viscosity. Warming the mastic in a pan of hot water will thin it and make it easier to measure.

Formula 1

     10 drops geranium essential oil
      3 drops thyme 'thujanol' essential oil
     ½ g mastic (a bead about the size of a pencil eraser)
     30 ml (1 ounce) apricot oil

Formula 2

      3 drops sandalwood essential oil
      3 drops pine essential oil
      3 drops vetiver essential oil
      1 g mastic (a bead about the size of a pea)
     60 ml (2 ounces) St.-John's-wort oil

Mix the ingredients in a 60 ml (2 ounce) bottle and shake well.
To use: Massage into the groin to relieve prostate pain and congestion.

OBTAINING MASTIC

Mastic is available from many essential oil suppliers, including Leydet Aromatics (see Resources).

Indian Prostate Massage Oil

In India, the essential oil tulsi *(Thymus serpyllum)* is used to promote prostate health.

    10 drops geranium essential oil
     3 drops tulsi essential oil
  30 ml (1 ounce) foraha

Mix the ingredients in a 30 ml (1 ounce) bottle and shake well.
To use: Massage into the groin to promote prostate health.

GENITAL WARTS

There are two types of genital warts. One type is found in the groin area, usually in the leg creases. These are benign and not troublesome beyond the fact that they are unsightly. The French call them rooster combs, for obvious reasons if you have ever seen them. They can often be completely removed by applying mugwort oil directly to the lesion with a cotton swab once a day for three days. Use a very small amount of oil and take care not to get the mugwort on the surrounding healthy skin.

The other type of genital wart occurs on the tip of the penis. It can be very painful and is also highly contagious, spread through sexual contact. To treat this type of wart with essential oils, you must use diluted oils. Place 2 drops of *Eucalyptus citriodora* and 2 drops of chamomile essential oil on a mirror or other impermeable surface, and dilute with an equal amount of aloe vera gel. Apply the dilution directly to the wart with a cotton swab once a day until the lesion is gone.

MALE TONIC

Thuja cedar is a very powerful essential oil that is considered to be a male tonic. It is taken in very small doses — no more than a drop or two a day — to promote healthy circulation, prostate health, vigor, and sexuality. But thuja is very high in deadly ketones, which accumulate in the liver. Because of this high ketone content, thuja should not be used carelessly, even as a topical application. And if you are considering the oral use of thuja as a tonic, you should do so only under the guidance of a physician or naturopath who is well versed in the use of essential oils.

MALE TONIC INHALATION

This safe and effective tonic inhalation is invigorating and stimulating to male hormone function. This same blend can be mixed with 60 ml (2 ounces) of almond oil to make an invigorating massage or bath oil.

6 drops *Pinus pinaster* essential oil
6 drops tea tree essential oil
2 drops savory essential oil

Combine the essential oils in a small vial and inhale the scent periodically throughout the day.

ENHANCING SENSUALITY

The pleasure of touch is an important aspect of lovemaking. One of my clients, a musician named Michael, recently confided, "I primarily use oils as a tool to create sensual moments, and to help keep me focused." Each of these blends will enhance the sensuality of mutual massage as a prelude to lovemaking.

SENSUAL MASSAGE OIL

Formula 1

    5 drops jasmine essential oil
    5 drops frankincense essential oil
    5 drops sandalwood essential oil
  60 ml (2 ounces) apricot oil

Formula 2

    2 drops cardamom essential oil
    5 drops jasmine essential oil
    5 drops sandalwood essential oil
    2 drops rose essential oil
  60 ml (2 ounces) apricot oil

Mix the ingredients in a 60 ml (2 ounce) bottle and shake well.

APHRODISIAC BATH

4 drops jasmine essential oil   4 drops neroli essential oil
4 drops ginger essential oil   6 drops clary sage
2 drops cumin essential oil   essential oil

Add the essential oils to a cup (235 ml) of milk or solubol and mix into a hot bath.

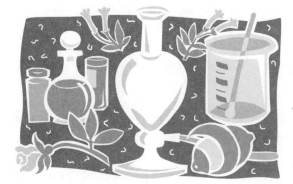

Aromatherapy for Successful Aging

People age at different rates, and although genetics play a big role in the aging process, it is important to remember that genes only indicate tendencies; they are not predictors of destiny. My main concern with aging is not so much old age itself but the increased risk of disease and disability that the condition entails. My goal is to maintain a healthy physical and mental function and a continued engagement in life. Although at this time there is no eternal fountain of youth, and antiaging potions mostly don't work, aromatherapy has a lot to offer an aging population. Aromatherapy can help keep the aging mind sharp and the spirit optimistic; it can work to protect the body's systems from the ravages of degenerative disease.

MAINTAINING CONFIDENCE

One of the most important markers for successful aging is confidence — confidence in your ability to perform activities in a functional manner. Although your intensity of activity and even your definition of functional performance may need to be adjusted and no doubt scaled down as you age, confidence in your abilities is a crucial factor in aging gracefully.

ADRENAL-STIMULATING DIFFUSER BLEND

Diffusing this blend in the home environment will perk up energy and help maintain motivation.

Formula 1
40 drops cedarwood essential oil
20 drops citronella essential oil
40 drops geranium essential oil

Formula 2

> 20 drops *Eucalyptus citriodora* essential oil
> 60 drops juniper essential oil
> 20 drops everlasting essential oil

Combine the essential oils in a diffuser and run for up to three hours per day.

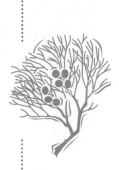

FRENCH FRAILTY TONIC

French phytotherapy literature identifies the essential oils cinnamon, angelica, oregano, and summer savory as particularly helpful in treating conditions of geriatric frailty. The following recipe is adapted from a popular French tonic.

> 2 drops cinnamon essential oil
> 2 drops angelica essential oil
> 2 drops oregano essential oil
> 2 drops savory essential oil
> 5 ml (1 teaspoon) solubol or honey
> 235 ml (1 cup) hot water

Dissolve the essential oils in the honey or solubol and stir into the hot water.

To use: Taken three times daily — at midday, early evening, and upon retiring — this tonic is believed to restore strength and vitality, particularly in cases in which muscular atrophy has occurred. In France, the formula is traditionally taken in red wine. (See caution regarding internal use on page 131.)

British Restorative Massage Oil

In Great Britain, basil is used in restorative massage therapy for bedridden geriatric patients.

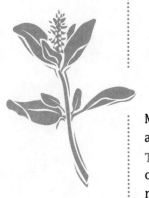

60 ml (2 ounces) olive or almond oil
12 drops lavender essential oil
12 drops rosemary essential oil
10 drops eucalyptus essential oil
6 drops basil essential oil

Measure the carrier oil into a 60 ml (2 ounce) dark glass bottle and add the essential oils; shake to mix.

To use: Massage to stimulate circulation and restore muscle tone, or as a body oil, around the elbows and knees especially, to promote circulation.

Promoting Physical Activity

The fear of old age is often the fear of becoming helpless and dependent on others for basic needs and care. We will all eventually need some assistance if we live long enough, and turning to others in a time of need is part of the human condition. Still, elderly independence can be prolonged substantially by maintaining a healthy level of physical activity. Restricted activity inevitably leads to a decline in physical strength, which increases the risk of falls, as well as the chance that a fall will result in a serious injury. Sedentary people of any age will benefit enormously from even the most minimal exercise program. Strength training improves balance and decreases falls remarkably.

The following blends are most beneficial as massage oils, used before or after a strength training session or other physical exertion. Each can also be added to the bath or used as a body oil.

LEG MASSAGE OIL

10 drops cypress essential oil
6 drops sage essential oil
10 drops lemon essential oil
30 ml (1 ounce) sesame oil

Blend the essential oils in the sesame oil and mix well.
To use: Massage tired or painful legs.

REJUVENATING BLEND

This blend will ease aches and pains and rejuvenate old bones and joints.

30 ml (1 ounce) sesame oil
30 ml (1 ounce) evening primrose or borage oil
3 drops clove essential oil
6 drops orange essential oil
6 drops lavender essential oil
3 drops camphor essential oil
6 drops eucalyptus essential oil
6 drops rosemary essential oil
2 drops peppermint essential oil

Blend the carrier oils in a 60 ml (2 ounce) dark glass bottle and add the essential oils; shake to mix.

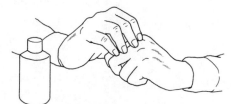

Regular aromatherapy massage can help relieve the pain of arthritic joints.

WARMING BLEND

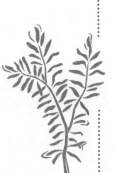

30 ml (1 ounce) flaxseed oil
30 ml (1 ounce) olive oil
60 ml (2 ounces) almond oil
 6 drops rosemary essential oil
 6 drops ginger essential oil
 6 drops benzoin essential oil
 6 drops black pepper essential oil
 6 drops cayenne essential oil

Blend the carrier oils in a 120 ml (4 ounce) dark glass bottle and add the essential oils; shake to mix.

To use: This blend will prepare arthritic joints for a session of strength training or other physical exertion. It will also ease aches and pains in cold weather.

COOLING BLEND

30 ml (1 ounce) flaxseed oil
30 ml (1 ounce) olive oil
60 ml (2 ounces) almond oil
10 drops birch essential oil
 2 drops peppermint essential oil
12 drops lavender essential oil
 3 drops everlasting essential oil

Blend the carrier oils in a 120 ml (4 ounce) dark glass bottle and add the essential oils; shake to mix.

To use: This formula is good to use following a strength-training session or other physical exertion to minimize muscle stiffness. It will also cool and relieve the pain of inflammatory arthritis.

HELPING THE BODY COMBAT AGING

Aging might be described as an accumulation of cellular damage, of toxins gumming up cellular transmitters and blocking chemical message sites. Most of this cellular damage is caused by free radicals.

Free radicals are injured cells, or particles of cells, that have become unstable oxygen molecules. They are the result of exposure to external irritants such as environmental pollution, radiation, electromagnetic waves, sunlight, harmful chemicals, food additives, tobacco smoke, and numerous other substances. Modern life bombards us with free-radical fuel on an hourly basis. Equally important is the action of our own body's metabolic process. Free radicals are produced in the body in reaction to infection and stress, and by our own fat metabolism.

Free radicals have unpaired electrons that cause them to seek connections with other molecules. In their quest to connect they penetrate healthy cells and damage the genetic material within. As this damage accumulates, our body's ability to combat aging, cancer, hardening of the arteries, arthritis, and other degenerative changes is drastically reduced. The wrinkles and brown spots, along with the bumps and blemishes and cancerous skin lesions, that we associate with old age are actually the visible manifestation of these damaged cells. Even though our body is able eliminate free radicals by using white blood cells, it taxes the resources of our immune system to do so. With the increasing amounts of free radicals in our bodies, more of our immune-system resources are spent cleaning up free radicals.

Antioxidants for a Strong Immune System

Antioxidants are a group of vitamins, minerals, enzymes, and essential oils that Mother Nature has provided to protect our genetic material from assaults by free radicals. The use of antioxidants to help combat free radicals frees up our immune system to identify and

SUPER-ANTIOXIDANT ESSENTIAL OILS

Clove
Fenugreek
Marjoram
Nutmeg
Oregano
Paprika
Pepper
Rosemary
Sage
Savory
Tarragon
Thyme

fight other enemies. Antioxidants latch onto free radicals in our body, forming a clump that can no longer penetrate healthy cells and that is easily eliminated as a waste product. The result is a healthier immune system and less cell damage. Among other things, antioxidants can help our systems resist infection and the degeneration of aging diseases. Unfortunately, most modern diets are lacking in sufficient antioxidants and supporting nutrients to counterbalance the overwhelming onslaught of free radicals on our biological system. Antioxidants have become one of the fastest-growing segments of the nutritional supplement market.

Essential fatty acids are important antioxidants that are abundantly present in flaxseed oil, sesame oil, evening primrose oil, and borage oil. These oils are particularly valuable for their antiaging properties and can be ingested as well as being used as carrier oils for massage and body oil blends.

Antioxidant Essential Oils

The essential oils thyme, sage, marjoram, oregano, rosemary, and savory have received a lot of attention in France for their antioxidant properties. Thyme is emerging as a worldwide favorite for its antiaging properties. In addition to its antioxidant properties, thyme acts as a very powerful bactericidal, as well as a stimulant to the immune system.

Studies conducted in Ireland have found the essential oils of clove, nutmeg, pepper, tarragon, fenugreek, and paprika to be effective free-radical scavengers. When these oils were added to the water supplies of laboratory rats, the animals' aging processes were measurably slowed down.

You can make your own daily antioxidant supplement by adding one or two drops of one of these antioxidant essential oils to a tablespoon of antioxidant carrier oil. Experiment with different oils and combinations to find one that agrees with you.

SUPER-ANTIOXIDANT CARRIER OILS

Borage
Evening primrose
Flaxseed
Sesame seed

DEMENTIA AND ALZHEIMER'S DISEASE

The term *dementia* describes a deterioration of mental faculties, including memory. Often referred to as the "second childhood," dementia robs its victims of their intellect and their independence. Often the most obvious symptom of Alzheimer's disease, dementia can also be the result of malnutrition, compromised circulation, or other conditions of aging. In the United States dementia affects approximately four million people. Due to increased life expectancy, the dementia population is predicted to quintuple by the year 2040.

A number of dementia treatments have been tried, ranging from drugs to high-pressure oxygen and psychostimulants, with disappointing results. Simple massage, however, with a formula of grapeseed oil, melissa, and lavender, rendered improved mobility, mental function, and communication as well as an increased desire to become active to dementia patients at a residential care facility in Great Britain.

Alzheimer's disease, one of the leading causes of dementia, is a progressive, degenerative, and eventually fatal disease that attacks the brain and results in impaired memory, thinking, and behavior. Alzheimer's patients become agitated and disorientated, often angry and obsessive. The disease afflicts many millions throughout the world and exacts a heavy toll, not only on the patient but also on the patient's family and friends. Conventional medicine has found little to treat this devastating disease. Modern medical research still has not discovered the primary causes of Alzheimer's disease, although the gallery of suspects ranges from genes to environmental toxins and viral infections.

The primary treatment for Alzheimer's patients is to provide emotional support and stability in a calm and safe environment. Often the patient is best served by providing support to the primary caregiver. In this case, calming and emotionally stabilizing oils and blends are indicated.

**DEMENTIA
MASSAGE OIL**

Blend 3 drops of melissa essential oil and 15 drops of lavender essential oil into 1 ounce (30 ml) of grapeseed oil. Use as a massage or body oil.

Lavender oil, diffused into the atmosphere of a residential care facility for Alzheimer's patients in Lodi, California, had very good results. The staff noted a marked decrease in agitation of specific patients and a much calmer mood in general throughout the facility.

Aromatherapy is a new frontier for successful aging and support of geriatric conditions. Essential oils are beginning to get attention from the scientific community. Hopefully that attention will inspire the initiation of aromatherapy programs in many more hospitals and residential care facilities.

MARGUERITE MAURY'S BLEND FOR AGING COUPLES

Dementia victims often become unreasonable and uncooperative, resisting the assistance of loved ones. This behavior can be particularly distressing to an equally aged spouse who is struggling to maintain his or her own health while caring for an unreasonable partner. Marguerite Maury, one of the pioneers of modern aromatherapy, recommended essential oils of lemongrass, rose, and black pepper to ease the conflicts faced by aging couples. She felt this combination would be particularly helpful to women who must deal with difficult old men.

3 drops lemongrass essential oil

5 drops rose essential oil

3 drops black pepper essential oil

30 ml (1 ounce) almond oil

Blend the essential oils in the almond oil and mix well.

To use: Apply as a massage or body oil. Without the almond oil, this blend can also be made into a clarifying inhalation. Mix the essential oils in a small vial. Place a drop on a cotton ball and waft the scent in front of both parties' faces to defuse moments of conflict or frustration.

Glossary

Absolute: The pure essential oil, extracted from a concrète through alcohol process

Actinic keratosis: Horny skin growth caused by exposure to ultraviolet light

Acupressure: Noninvasive body work that acts on the traditional meridians of the body

Acupuncture: Traditional Chinese practice of piercing with needles at specific sites to treat disease or relieve pain

Adrenal cortex: The part of the adrenal gland that produces a variety of steroid hormones

Alchemy: An early form of chemistry with philosophic and magical associations

Alcohol: A class of organic compounds that contain one or more hydroxyl groups (OH) and react with acids to form esters

Aldehyde: A class of organic compounds that contain the CHO group

Alembic: Anything that refines or purifies by distillation

Allopathic medicine: A philosophy of medicine that treats disease by using remedies that produce an opposite effect of that produced by disease

Analgesic: Pain masking

Anticatarrhal: Minimizes or prevents inflammation of a mucous membrane

Anticoagulant: Minimizes or prevents the coagulant action of blood

Antidepressant: Minimizes or prevents depression

Antifungal: Minimizes or prevents overgrowth of fungus

Antigenic: A substance to which the body reacts by producing antibodies

Antihistamine: Minimizes or prevents the actions of hitamine, as in an allergic reaction

Antimicrobial: Able to inhibit or control microbes

Antioxidant: A substance that slows the oxidation of hydrocarbons, thus checks deterioration

Antipigmentary: Minimizes or prevents the discoloration of skin associated with damage and age

Antirheumatic: Minimizes or prevents various types of pain in the joints and muscles

Antiseptic: Inhibits the actions of microorganisms

Antispasmodic: Relieving or preventing spasms

Antiviral: Capable of checking the growth of a virus

Aperitif: Appetite stimulant

Apocrine gland: Specialized gland that secretes highly scented cellular detritus along with clear sweat

Arteriosclerosis: Abnormal thickening and loss of elasticity in the walls of the arteries

Astringent: Contracts body tissue

Auric field: The confines of the visible emanation surrounding a physical body

Auro soma: A system of color, crystals, herbs & essential oils developed by Vicky Wall

Autonomic nervous system: The part of the nervous system that is responsible for control and regulation of involuntary bodily functions

Ayurveda: Traditional Hindu medicine

Bactericidal: Possesses the ability to destroy bacteria

Balneotherapy: Therapeutic bathing

Base oil: Same as carrier oil, used to dilute, carry, and deliver essential oils

Bass note: In perfumery, the foundation, the least volatile scent in a blend

Benzene: A toxic aromatic liquid obtained through the distillation of coal tar

Beta-carotene: A precursor to the production of vitamin A in the liver

Bile: A bitter alkaline bodily humor that aids in digestion

Bolus: Aka ovule, a vaginal suppository

Breathwork: The practice of controlled breathing for health and meditation purposes

Carminative: Causing gas to be expelled from the stomach and intestines

Carotenoid: Any of several red and yellow plant and animal pigments

Carrier oil: Same as base oil, used to dilute, carry, and deliver essential oils

Catalyst: A substance serving as an agent in a chemical reaction

Chakra: One of the seven body centers considered to be the source of spiritual energy

Chemotype: A composition of the essential oil in which one chemical dominates over the norm

Chi: Vital energy

Chypre: A classification of perfume, chypres share a common theme in their bass of oakmoss, patchouli, and amber, combined with a fresh citrusy top note

Cold extraction: A method of extracting essential oils from plant material without the use of heat

Cold process: Oils processed under 280 degrees are considered to be cold process

Colitis: Inflammation of the large intestine

Colloidal mineral supplement: Colloidal mineral particles are small enough to remain suspended in liquid or gas but, unlike dissolved particles, retain their whole form

Color therapy: The use of colored lights or gels (theatrical lighting colored acetate sheets) for healing

Concrète: A compound of fat and essential oils, the product of enfleurage

Contusion: A bruise or injury in which the skin is not broken

Counterirritant: Anything used to produce a slight irritation, in order to relieve more serious inflammation elsewhere

Critical carbon dioxide: Refers to a process of extracting essential oils at a subfreezing temperature

Cystitis: Inflammation of the urinary bladder

Deep tissue work: A special form of massage that uses deep pressure and works to release tension and congestion held in the muscles and deeper tissue

Dermatitis: Inflammation of the skin

DHEA: A steroidal hormone that peaks in early adulthood and declines rapidly with age

Diluent: A diluting substance

Diosgenin: A steroid found in yams

Diuretic: Increasing the excretion of urine

Dosha: An Ayurvedic term referring to a constitutional type or description of a set of physical and emotional patterns

Duodenum: The first section of the small intestine

Eczema: A noncontagious skin disorder characterized by inflammation, itching, and scales

Edema: An abnormal accumulation of fluids in the cells, tissues, or cavities of the body

Electron: An elementary particle, part of an atom that holds a negative charge

Emollient: Something that has a softening or soothing effect

Emulsifier: A substance that enables one liquid to be dispersed and suspended in another without dissolving

Endocrine: Of any hormone-producing gland

Endometriosis: The growth of endometrial (uterine lining) tissue in abnormal locations

Endorphin: A pain-relieving substance secreted in the brain

Enfleurage: A method of extracting essential oils by absorbing them with fat

Enzyme: An organic catalyst to chemical reactions

Epidermis: The outermost layer of the skin

Essential fatty acid: One of a family of molecules that are essential to the health of, but not manufactured by, the human body and must be obtained from outside sources

Ester: A fruity smelling molecule found in beer, wine, and certain esssential oils

Estrogen: A hormone produced in the ovaries and responsible for many bodily functions

Ether: A molecule that has a unique licorice-like odor

Excipient: An inert substance added to a formula to acheive a desired consistency or form

Exfoliate: To remove surface skin and dead skin cells

Expectorant: A substance that encourages the expression of mucus from the throat and lungs through coughing

Fatty acid: A type of naturally occurring lipid that appears in animal and vegetable fats and oils

Fibrocystic breast: The ocurrence of benign fibrous growths in the breast tissue

Fixative: A substance that prevents or minimizes fading of scent

Fixed oil: Not volatile

Florasol: Also phytol, a product of the phytonic process

Free radical: An atom or molecule having at least one unpaired electron, usually reactive and unstable

Fumigant: Any substance used to create fumes

Functional group: A special arrangement of atoms in a molecule that is subject to a characteristic chemical behavior

Genus: A group of closely related species

Glycerin: An odorless, colorless, syrupy liquid

Hematoma: A collection of blood, usually clotted, under the skin

Hemostatic: Encourages coagulation of blood

Hepatic: Of or affecting the liver

Holistic: Dealing with the body as an integrated system, rather than with separate parts

Homeopathy: A philosophy of medicine that treats disease by using remedies that produce a similar effect to that of disease

Humectant: A substance added or applied to another to help it retain moisture

Hydrosol: A by-product of steam distillation, created as the water becomes impregnated with the aroma of the plant being distilled

Hyperallergenic: More than normally susceptible to allergens

Hypertension: Abnormally high blood pressure

Hypotension: Abnormally low blood pressure

Impetigo: A bacterial skin disease

Infusion: The liquid extract that results from steeping a substance in oil or water

Insulin: A hormone, produced by the pancreas, that metabolizes sugar and carbohydrates

Ion: An electrically charged atom or group of atoms

Isoprene: A branched structure composed of five carbon atoms, onto which hydrogen can easily bond

Kapha: A constitutional classification in Ayurvedic medicine

Keloid: An excessive growth of scar tissue on the skin

Ketone: An organic chemical compound; as a constituent in essential oils ketones are toxic, powerful, and aggressive

Kinesiology: Testing the muscles of the body to get information from the body

Laryngitis: Inflammation of the larynx, characterized by hoarseness or loss of voice

Lipid: Any of a group of organic compounds that are insoluble in water, and soluble in fat solvents and alcohols

Lymphatic: Of, containing, or conveying lumph

Lytic: Causing a dissolution or decomposition

Maceration: To soften and break down by squeezing and soaking

Medulla oblongata: The lowest portion of the brain, controls breathing and circulation

Meridian: The electromagnetic nerve channels that run through the body

Metaphysics: The study of the paranormal

Middle note: The theme, or heart note of a perfume blend

Monoterpene: A molecule composed of two isoprene units, or ten carbon atoms joined head to tail

Mucolytic: A substance that thins mucus, making it easier to eliminate from the lungs and bronchials

Naturopathy: A system of treating disease that uses natural elements and rejects the use of most drugs and medicines

Nebulizer: A pump that reduces a liquid to a very fine mist

Nervine: Calming to the nervous system

Neuralgia: Pain along the course of a nerve

Neurotoxin: A toxin that destroys nerves or nervous tissue

Organic chemistry: The branch of chemistry dealing with carbon compounds

Orthobionomy: A gentle alignment of bones through positioning and soft tissue release

Osteopathy: A system of medicine placing special emphasis on the relation of the musculoskeletal system to all other body systems

Osteoporosis: A bone disorder characterized by a reduction in bone density and an increase in brittleness and porosity

Ovule: Also bolus, a vaginal suppository

Oxidation: A chemical reaction in which oxygen combines with another substance, as in burning or rust

Parasympathetic nervous system: That part of the autonomic nervous system that opposes the sympathetic nervous system and regulates various responses such as a slowed heartbeat and constriction of the pupils of the eyes

pH: The degree of acidity or alkalinity of a solution

Phenol: An organic molecule, similar to alcohol, in essential oils; bactericidal and subject to oxidation

Phenyl: A molecular base for many aromatic compounds

Pheromone: A chemical substance secreted by animals and insects that conveys information and produces specific responses in other individuals of the same species

Phlebitis: Inflammation of a vein

Phytoestrogen: A substance from plant sources that is interpreted as an estrogen by human metabolism

Phytol: The resulting essential oil product of the phytonic process

Phytonic process: A method of plant oil extraction

Phytotherapy: Plant based medicine

Pineal gland: A small glandular outgrowth of the brain that produces the hormone melatonin

Pitta: A constitutional classification in Ayurvedic medicine

Pituitary gland: A small endocrine gland attached to the base of the brain that produces various hormones influencing growth, metabolism, and other endocrine activity

Pneuma: The soul or spirit

Polyunsaturated fat: A fat containing more than one double or triple bond in the molecule

Polyvalent: Having many uses

Pomade: A perfumed ointment

Poultice: A hot, moist mass applied to an inflamed or injured part of the body

Prikriti: In Ayurvedic theory, the unique combination of qualities that comprise an individual's constitution

Progesterone: A steroid hormone, active in preparing the uterus for the reception and development of a fertilized egg

Propolis: A waxy substance collected by bees from the buds of certain trees

Prostaglandin: Hormonelike fatty acids found throughout the body that affect important body processes

Psoriasis: A chronic skin disease characterized by scaly, red patches

Psychostimulant: Stimulating to the mind

Pulmonary: Of, like, or affecting the lungs

Pulse point: A point on the body where the pulse can be felt

Radiesthesia: The art of pendulum dowsing

Reflexology: Treating and diagnosing ailments through pressue and massage to corresponding areas on the foot, hand, and ear

Resin: A solid or semisolid substance exuded from various plants or trees

Sacrum: The thick, triangular bone at the lower end of the spinal column that forms the dorsal part of the pelvis

Saturated fat: A fat that remains solid at room temperature

Scabies: A parasitic skin mite

Sciatica: Inflammation of the sciatic nerve, the long nerve passing down the back of the thigh

Scleroderma: A hardening and thickening of the skin due to abnormal fibrous tissue growth

Sebaceous gland: A skin gland that secretes sebum

Sebum: A semiliquid greasy skin secretion

Seratonin: A neurotransmitter and hormone

Sesquiterpene: A molecule with three isoprene units, or 15 carbon atoms joined together head to tail

Shen point: An integration point located on the ear, considered an important access point to the brain

Shiatsu: A system of applying thumb pressure to acupressure points on the body

Shingles: A manifestation of the herpes zoster virus characterized by inflamed, painful nerve endings around the trunk

Silica: A hard glassy mineral found in a variety of forms

Skin tag: A small fleshy benign growth

Solvent: A substance that can dissolve another substance

Species: A naturally existing population of similar organisms that usually interbreed only among themselves

Stomachic: Digestive tonic

Subcutaneous: Beneath the skin

Symbology: The study, or interpretation, of symbols

Sympathetic nervous system: That part of the autonomic nervous system that stimulates the body to prepare for physical action or emergency

Synergism: The simultaneous action of separate agents that together have a greater impact that the sum of their individual effects

Systemic: Affecting the entire organism

Taxonomy: The science of classification

Temporal limbic: A primitive part of the brain

Terpene: A molecule made up of carbon and hydrogen atoms

Terpineol: Any of three isomeric alcohols with a lilac odor

Terroir: A French word that means the expression of the earth, or the particular planting site, in the resultant essential oil; a factor of soil, shade, wind, water, rain, and terrain

Thalassotherapy: Bath therapy using seawater or plants

Therapeutic Touch: Modern energy transfer therapy most often practiced by nurses

Third Eye: The sixth chakra, a clairvoyant center located between the eyes

Thrombosis: A blood clot in the heart or a blood vessel

Tonic: Invigorating or stimulating

Top note: The first and most fleeting scent in a perfume blend

Touch for Health: A system developed by John Thie that combines applied kinesiology for a diagnosis and acupressure touch for treating the musculoskeletal system

Transdermal: To pass through the skin

Tridoshic: In Ayurvedic theory, a constitution composed equally of the three doshas

Trigger point: A point on the body that, when stimulated, affects other areas of the body

Unsaturated fat: A fat that remains liquid at room temperature

Vascular: Having to do with the blood vessels

Vata: A constitutional classification in Ayurvedic medicine

Vicosity: The relative fluidity of a liquid

Volatile: Having a tendency to vaporize or evaporate quickly

Bibliography

Abehsera, Michael. *The Clay Book.* Secaucus, NJ: Citadel, 1977.

Arctander, Steffen. *Perfume and Flavor Materials of Natural Origin.* Elizabeth, NJ: self-published, 1960.

Avery, Alexandra. *Aromatherapy and You.* Birkenfeld, OR: Blue Heron Hill Press, 1992.

Bernadet, Marcel. *Phytotherapie.* St-Jean-de-Braye, France: Editions Dangles, 1983.

Berwick, Ann. *Holistic Aromatherapy.* St. Paul, MN: Llewellyn, 1994.

Bolen, Jean Shinoda. *Goddesses in Every Woman.* New York: Harper & Row, 1985.

Corbin, Alain. *The Foul and the Fragrant.* Cambridge, MA: Harvard University Press, 1986.

Chopra, Deepak. *Perfect Health.* New York: Harmony Books, 1991.

Cunningham, Scott. *Magical Aromatherapy.* St. Paul, MN: Llewellyn, 1989.

———. *The Magic of Incense Oils and Brews.* St. Paul, MN: Llewelyn, 1986.

Davis, Patricia. *Aromatherapy A–Z.* Saffron, Essex, England: C. W. Daniel Co., 1988.

———. *Subtle Aromatherapy.* Saffron, Essex, England: C. W. Daniel Co. 1989.

Dextreit, Raymond. *Our Earth, Our Cure.* Brooklyn, NY: Swan House, 1974.

Dodt, Colleen. *The Essential Oil Book.* Pownal, VT: Storey Publishing, 1994.

Dye, Jane. *Aromatherapy for Women and Children.* Saffron, Essex, England: C. W. Daniel Co., 1992.

Edwards, Victoria. *Aromatherapy Blue Chart.* Fair Oaks, CA: self-published, 1990.

England, A. *Aromatherapy for Mother and Baby.* Rochester, VT: Healing Arts Press, 1994.

Fischer-Rizzi, Suzanne. *Complete Aromatherapy Handbook.* New York: Sterling, 1990.

Gattefossé, Rene Maurice. *Aromatherapie.* Paris, France: Giradot & Cie Librairie des Sciences, 1937; reprint, San Francisco: S. F. Herbal Studies Library, 1990.

Greer, Mary. *The Essence of Magic.* North Hollywood, CA: Newcastle, 1993.

Grosjean, Nelly. *Aromatherapy from Provence.* Saffron, Essex, England: C. W. Daniel Co., 1994

———. *Veterinary Aromatherapy* Essex, England: C. W. Daniel Co., 1994.

Guenther, E. *The Essential Oils.* New York: Van Nostrand, 1948.

Gumbel, Dietrich. *Principles of Holistic Skin Care with Herbal Essences.* Heidelburg: Haug, 1986.

Gurudas. *Flower Essences.* Albuquerque: Brotherhood of Life, Inc., 1983.

Hephrun, Bernie. *Essential Oils and Aromatherapy.* London: self-published, 1989.

Haarmann & Reimer. *Fragrance Guide. Fragrances on the International Market.* Hamburg, Germany: H & R Perfume Books, Verlagsgesellschaft R. Gloess & Co., 1989.

Irvine, Susan. *Perfume.* Avenel, NJ: Crescent, 1995.

Junneman, Monika. *Enchanting Scents.* Wilot, WI: Lotus Light Publications, 1988.

Junemann, Monika, and Maggie Tisserand. *The Magic and Power of Lavender.* Essex, England: C. W. Daniel Co., 1998.

Keville, Kathi. *Pocket Guide to Aromatherapy.* Freedom, CA: Crossing Press, 1996.

Keville, Kathi, and Mindy Green. *Aromatherapy: A Complete Guide.* Freedom, CA: Crossing Press, 1995.

Lautie, R., and A. Passebecq. *Aromatherapy: The Use of Plant Essences in Healing.* Wellingborough, England: Thorsons, 1979.

Lavabre, Marcel. *The Aromatherapy Workbook.* Rochester, VT: Healing Arts Press, 1990.

Lawless, Julia. *Aromatherapy and the Mind.* Wellingborough, England: Thorsons, 1998.

———. *Encyclopedia of Essential Oils.* New York: Element Books, 1995.

———. *The Illustrated Encyclopedia of Essential Oils.* New York: Element Books, 1995.

Leon, Vicki. *Uppity Women of Ancient Times.* Berkeley, CA: Conari Press, 1995.

Mabberley, D. J. *The Plant Book.* 2nd ed. Cambridge: Cambridge University Press, 1997.

Mailhebiau, Philippe. *Portraits in Oils.* Essex, England: C. W. Daniel Co., 1995.

Maple, Eric. *The Magic of Perfume.* New York: Samuel Weiser, 1973.

Maury, Marguerite. *How to Dowse.* London, England: British Society of Dowsers, 1953.

———. *The Secret of Life and Youth.* London, England: Dorling Kindersley, Ltd., 1964.

Maxwell-Hudson, Clare. *Aromatherapy Massage.* London: DK, 1994.

Miller, Dr. Light, and Bryan Miller. *Ayurveda and Aromatherapy.* Twin Lakes, WI: Lotus Press, 1996.

Miller, Richard. *Magical and Ritual Use of Perfumes.* Rochester, VT: Destiny Books, 1988.

Morris, Edwin T. *Fragrance: The Story of Perfume from Cleopatra to Chanel.* New York: Scribner, 1984.

Northrup, Christiane. *Women's Bodies, Women's Wisdom.* New York: Bantam Doubleday Dell, 1994.

Packard, Candis Cantin. *Pocket Guide to Ayurvedic Healing.* Freedom, CA: Crossing Press, 1996.

Paltz, Jacques. *Le Fascinant pouvoir des huiles essentielles.* Paris: self-published, 1984.

Paravati, Jeanne. *Hygeia: A Woman's Herbal.* San Francisco: Freestone, 1978.

Penoel, Daniel, and P. Franchomme. *Aromatherapie exactement.* Limoges, France: Roger Jollois, 1990.

Perry, Rachel. *Reverse the Aging Process of Your Face.* New York: Dell, 1984.

Price, Shirley. *Practical Aromatherapy.* Wellingborough, England: Thorsons, 1983.

———. *Aromatherapy Workbook.* Wellingborough, England: Thorsons, 1993.

Prince, Menkit. *The Essential Oil Cookbook.* Carmichael, CA: Self-published, 1998.

Robbins, Tom. *Jitterbug Perfume.* New York: Bantam Books, 1990.

Rose, Jeanne. *The Aromatherapy Book: Applications and Inhalations.* Berkeley, CA: North Atlantic, 1992.

———. *Herbs and Things.* New York: Grosset & Dunlap, 1974.

———. *Herbs for the Reproductive System.* Berkeley, CA: Frog, Ltd., 1994.

———. *375 Essential Oils and Hydrosols.* Berkeley, CA: North Atlantic, 1999.

Rose, Jeanne, and Susan Earle, eds. *World of Aromatherapy.* Berkeley, CA: North Atlantic, 1996.

Ryman, Danielle. *Aromatherapy Handbook.* Saffron Walde, England: C.W. Daniel Co,, 1984.

———. *Aromatherapy: The Complete Guide.* New York: Bantam, 1991.

Schnaubelt, Kurt. *Advanced Aromatherapy.* Rochester, VT: Healing Arts Press, 1998.

———. *Aromatherapy Course.* San Rafael, CA: self-published, 1984.

———. *Medical Aromatherapy.* Berkeley, CA: North Atlantic Books, 1992.

Treben, Maria. *God's Pharmacy.* Emmsthaler, Austria: Steyr, Wilhelm, 1980.

Tisserand, Maggie. *Aromatherapy for Women.* Northhamptonshire, England: Thorsons, 1985.

Tisserand, Robert. *Art of Aromatherapy.* Rochester, VT: Inner Traditions, 1988.

Tisserand, Robert, and Tony Balacs. *Essential Oil Safety Data Manual.* Brighton, England: Association of Tisserand Aromatherapists, 1985.

Valnet, Jean. *Practice of Aromatherapy.* New York: Destiny, 1982.

Wall, V. *Miracle of Color Healing.* Wellingborough, England: Thorsons, 1993.

Weed, Susan. *Menopausal Years.* Woodstock, NY: Ash Tree, 1989.

Westwood, C. *Aromatherapy: A Guide for Home Use.* Dorset, England: Amberwood Publishing, 1991.

White, Judith. *Aromatherapy for Lovers and Dreamers.* New York: Crown, 1996.

Wildwood, C. *Aromatherapy Massage with Essential Oils.* New York: Barnes & Noble, 1991 (out of print).

Williams, D. *The Chemistry of Essential Oils.* Dorset, England: Michelle Press, 1996.

Worwood, Valerie. *Aromantics.* London: Cavaye Place Pan Books, 1987.

———. *Complete Book of Essential Oils.* Novato, CA: New World Library, 1991.

———. *Fragrant Mind.* Novato, CA: New World Library, 1996.

———. *The Fragrant Pharmacy.* London: Macmillan, 1990.

Periodical, Journal, & Magazine Articles

Edwards, V. "Synthetic and Natural Oils." *International Journal of Aromatherapy (IJA)* 2, no. 2 (1989).

———. "A Rose Is a Rose." *Common Scents* (AATA) 1, no. 2–3 (1988–1989).

———. "Aroma Points." *Scentsitivity* (NAHA) 1, no. 4 (1996).

———. "Emotional Chart." *Scentsitivity* (NAHA) 1, no. 6 (1996).

Graham, Joy. "Inula." Self-published research paper, 1998.

Hobbs, Christopher. "St.-John's-Wort." *Let's Live* 5 (1995).

Kusmirek, J. "Carrier Oils." *International Federation of Aromatherapy Newsletter* 2, no. 8 (1989).

Mitchell, Stewart. "Dementia." *International Journal of Aromatherapy (IJA)* 5, no. 2 (1993).

Rose, Jeanne. "A Short Course in Aromatherapy Botany" in *The Herbal Rose Report* and *Aromatherapy* (Fall 1998).

Scott, Christine. "In Profile: Jean Valnet." *International Journal of Aromatherapy (IJA)* 5, no. 4 (1994).

Striecher, C. "Everlast." *Scentsitivity* (NAHA) 8, no. 1 (1998).

Wilkenfeld, Irene. "Perfumery or Pollution?" *Green Alternatives* 32 (1992).

Resources

Associations

National Association of Holistic Aromatherapists
P.O. Box 17622
Boulder, CO 80308
(888) ASK-NAHA
info@naha.org

Canadian Federation of Aromatherapists
439 Wellington Street West
Toronto, Ontario M5V 1E7
(888) 578-7815
(416) 591-0270
(888) 340-4445
CICA@aromashoppe.com

International Federation of Aromatherapists
Stamford House
2–4 Chiswick High Road
London W4 1TH England
44-181-742-2605

Education

Aromatherapy Institute & Research/AIR
P.O. Box 2354
Fair Oaks, CA 95628
(916) 965-7546
leydet@leydet.com

Australasian College of Botanical Studies
P.O. Box 57
Lake Oswego, OR 97034
(800) 487-8839
www.herbed.com

Evergreen Herb Garden & School of Integrative Herbology
P.O. Box 1445
Placerville, CA 95667
(530) 626-9288
evrgreen@innercite.com

Rocky Mountain Center for Botanical Studies
c/o Mindy Green
Boulder, CO 80308-2254
(303) 447-9662

Oak Valley Herb Farm
c/o Kathy Keville
P.O. Box 2482
Nevada City, CA 95959

Jeanne Rose Aromatherapy
Lectures and seminars
219 Carl Street
San Francisco, CA 94117
(415) 564-6785

Amrita
c/o Christoph Streicher
1900 West Stone Avenue
Fairfield, IA 52556
(515) 472-9136

Aromatic Plant Project
219 Carl Street
San Francisco, CA 94117
www.aromaticplantproject.com

PIA
Kurt Schnaubelt
P.O. Box 6723
San Rafael, CA 94903

College of Botanical Healing Arts
c/o Elizabeth Van Buren
P.O. Box 7542
Santa Cruz, CA 95061
(831) 462-1807

Atlantic Institute of Aromatherapy
16018 Saddlestring Drive
Tampa, FL 33618
(813) 265-2222

Essential Oils

Leydet Aromatics
PO Box 2354
Fair Oaks, CA 95628
(916) 965-7546
leydet.com

Urban Herbalist
1729 L Street
Sacramento, CA 95814
(916) 447-HERB

Psycheology
3008 Chippewa
Prescott, AZ 86301
(520) 778-6951

Earthbound
529 South Street
Philadelphia, PA 19147
(215) 627-1797
www.ebound.com

Liberty Natural Products
8120 SE Stark Street
Portland, OR 97215
(503) 256-1227
(800) 289-8247
www.libertynatural.com

Mountain Herbs
466 Main Street
Placerville, CA 95667
(530) 621-4372

A Touch of Heaven
77–6420 Kilohana
Maui, HI 96740
(808) 331-1936
alohasherry@juno.com

Self Heal Herbs
1106 Blanshard Street
Victoria, BC V8W 2H6
Canada
(250) 383-1913
angelina@netcom.ca

Lhasa Karnak Herb Co.
2513 Telegraph Avenue
Berkeley, CA 94704
(510) 548-0380

Elizabeth Van Buren Aromatherapy
P.O. Box 7542
Santa Cruz, CA 95061
(800) 710-7759

Soaps

Plantlife, Inc.
11440 Sunrise Gold Circle,
Suite #14
Rancho Cordova, CA
95742-6594
(916) 851-1155
www.plantlife.net

Candles and Soaps

Moon and Stars
44139 Tyler Road
Belleville, MI 48111
(734) 697 1206
koiekan@provide.net

Bottles

Sunburst Bottle Co.
5710 Auburn Blvd. #7
Sacramento, CA 95841
(916) 348-5576
Sunburst@cwo.com

Carrier Oils

Janca's Jojoba Oil & Seed Company
456 East Juanita
Avenue #7
Mesa, AZ 85204
JANCAS3@aol.com

Index

Page numbers in *italics* indicate illustrations. Page numbers in **boldface** indicate charts. Entries in **boldface** indicate recipes.

Other Storey Books You Will Enjoy

The Candlemaker's Companion, by Betty Oppenheimer. Handmade candles are now easier to create than ever before with the illustrated step-by-step instructions in this book. Readers will learn how to create rolled, poured, molded, and dipped candles; scent, color, and decorate candles naturally; make luminaria, lanterns, and floating candles; and use specialty techniques like overdipping, painting, layering, and sculpting. 176 pages. Paperback. ISBN 0-88266-994-X.

Creating Fairy Garden Fragrances, by Linda K. Gannon. This beautifully illustrated book explores the magical, aromatic world of herbs and flowers and provides recipes for richly scented, exotic potpourri blends. Accompanying each blend are fairy and herbal lore, poetry, stories about the seasons, and gift packaging ideas. 64 pages. Hardcover. ISBN 1-58017-076-5.

The Essential Oils Book, by Colleen K. Dodt. A rich resource on the many applications of aromatherapy and its uses in everyday life, including aromas for the home, scents for business environments, and essences for the elderly. 160 pages. Paperback. ISBN 0-88266-913-3.

The Herbal Body Book, by Stephanie Tourles. Learn how to transform common herbs, fruits, and grains into safe, economical, and natural personal care items. Contains over 100 recipes to make facial scrubs, hair rinses, shampoos, soaps, cleansing lotions, moisturizers, lip balms, toothpaste, powders, insect repellent, and more. 128 pages. Paperback. ISBN 10-88266-880-3.

The Herbal Home Spa, by Greta Breedlove. These easy-to-make recipes include facial steams, scrubs, masks, and lip balms; massage oils, baths, rubs, and wraps; hand, nail, and foot treatments; and shampoos, dyes, and conditioners. Relaxing bathing rituals and massage techniques are also covered. 208 pages. Paperback. ISBN 0-88266-005-6.

Making Herbal Dream Pillows, by Jim Long. This lavishly illustrated book offers step-by-step instructions for creating 15 herbal dream pillows for custom-made dreams. Author Jim Long also explores the history of dream pillows and their ties to folk medicine and herbal mythology. 64 pages. Hardcover. ISBN 1-58017-075-7.

Perfumes, Splashes & Colognes, by Nancy M. Booth. A professional perfumer reveals her trade secrets for creating personalized scents and re-creating favorite perfumes using herbs, oils, and alcohol. 176 pages. Paperback. ISBN 0-88266-985-0.

The Soapmaker's Companion, by Susan Miller Cavitch. The most authoritative guide to making natural, vegetable-based soaps ever written. In addition to basic soapmaking instruction, readers will learn how to use specialty techniques like marbling, layering, and making transparent, liquid, and imprinted soaps. Includes information on chemistry, ingredients, additives, colorants, scents, and experimenting with fats and oils. 288 pages. Paperback. ISBN 0-88266-965-6.

These books and other Storey books are available at your bookstore, farm store, garden center, or directly from Storey Publishing, 210 MASS MoCA Way, North Adams, MA 01247, or by calling 1-800-441-5700. Or visit our Web site at www.storey.com.